THE
LACTOSE-FREE
FAMILY
COOKBOOK

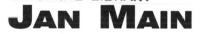
JAN MAIN

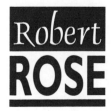

Original Canadian edition published in 1996 by
MacMillan Canada, Toronto.
Text Design: Page Active

Cataloguing information is located on page vi.

Cover Design: Matthews Communications Design
Photography: Mark Shapiro
Art Direction: Sharon Matthews
Food Stylist: Kate Bush
Prop Stylist: Charlene Ericson
Cover photo: Creamy Leek and Tomato Pasta. *page 90*

Distributed in the U.S. by
Firefly Books (U.S.) Inc.
P.O. Box 1338 Ellicott Station
Buffalo, NY 14205

Order Lines:
(416) 499-8412 voice
(416) 499-8313 fax

Published by Robert Rose Inc.
156 Duncan Mill Road, Suite 12
Toronto, Canada M3B 2N2
(416) 449-3535

Printed and bound in Canada

Contents

To my food friends
and to Rhoda,
whose enduring support spurred me on

Preface

For the lactose-intolerant individual, the experience of enjoying delicious meals without a tell-tale rumble from their tummy can be a rare event. They can't imagine sitting down to eat without having to have at least some special foods, as well as having to pass on tempting dishes reserved for others.

The *Lactose-Free Family Cookbook* ends this isolation. Jan Main has selected recipes that for years have been forbidden territory for many people with lactose intolerance. Cream soups, salmon mousse, béchamel sauce, rice pudding, cheesecake, tiramisu and ice creams are just a few of the delights that have been off-limits in the past.

This is not a textbook on living a lactose-free life. Instead, it is a beautifully written and well presented guidebook to tasty, healthy food that lactose-intolerant people can enjoy. The topic has been carefully researched in order to find substitutions that not only eliminate or substantially reduce lactose levels, but also provide additional health benefits. The reader gets a chance to increase knowledge of the importance of calcium in the diet and learn what will and will not work to enhance the supply of that mineral to the body. Thus the introduction and use of tofu (prepared with calcium salts) to enhance the calcium content of a recipe. This is definitely a plus for lactose-intolerant people since even though there are good dairy choices available, they are often rejected for fear of an adverse reaction.

The numerous tips and hints provided will benefit cooks of all abilities. The introduction provides useful information on tofu and soy milk—possibly new ingredients in a cook's repertoire. Lactose-reduced milk is also utilized, and is perhaps introduced to some for the first time.

The *Lactose-Free Family Cookbook* is a welcome addition to the kitchen libraries of people with lactose intolerance and others who enjoy tasty, interesting food.

MARSHA ROSEN, RD

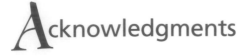cknowledgments

A book is never written in isolation. There are a number of people whose help, enthusiasm and interest were a tremendous inspiration and kept me at it.

- my students who first planted the seed of writing a cookbook
- Khristina Weinacht, lactose intolerant herself, who suggested the topic
- Janice Daciuk whose dietetic background, love of baking and organizational skills made testing recipes a joy
- Marsha Rosen for her gracious support
- Lesleigh Landry, Sandy Spurgeon and Lucy Gray for their testing competence
- my friends and family who critique the successes with the failures
- Kathy Johnson whose loving care of Alexa put my mind at rest

There are many more thank you's to be said, but to those people I give a personal thank you so this may remain succinct.

Canadian Cataloguing in Publication Data

Main, Jan

    The lactose-free family cookbook

U.S. ed.

Includes Index.

ISBN 1-896503-24-1

1. Milk-free diet - Recipes. I. Title

RM234.5.M35 1996   641.5'63   C96-930667-9

Introduction

In this book you will find recipes for all meals and every occasion suitable for friends and family to enjoy regardless of their tolerance to milk. My goal was to produce lactose-free recipes that taste great!

Recipes included are of two types:

* those based on milk that have been re-vamped with lactose-free soy foods, lactose-reduced milk, fruit juice and stock
* those that make a significant contribution to calcium.

Many people ask me if I am lactose intolerant and hence my interest in this topic. No, I am not, at least not at this point, but I do have an array of inconvenient food allergies, which makes me sympathetic to the cause. My friend Christina, newly diagnosed with lactose intolerance, suggested I write this cookbook to help her. It made sense as I began to understand her predicament. Christina is a wonderful cook of Hungarian background. She loved making cream-filled tortes, creamy sauces and cheese dishes. You can imagine her frustration. Even a drop of milk in her cup of tea caused discomfort.

At this time, I was teaching a cooking class to a Chinese group, all lactose intolerant. They have been excellent teachers to me! At one of our first classes we did a Koubiac of Salmon, always popular with past classes. I observed with some concern and wonder as the women happily tucked into the asparagus salad, gobbled down the Atlantic salmon with the wild rice and mushroom stuffing, ate sparingly of the green mayonnaise, and only tasted the flaky, buttery pastry that enveloped the salmon. My first lesson. The rich foods with sour cream and butter caused this lactose-intolerant group digestive problems.

Tofu was my next lesson. This same group introduced me to their tofu, superior to the tofu of my experience from a supermarket vegetable counter. This tofu had a delicate flavor and texture; in fact, it reminded me of custard. They told me how to care for tofu and different ways to prepare it. All news to me. Five pounds of tofu can go a long way in recipe experimentation! When I discovered that in addition to the creamy texture tofu gave to dishes, it was also a calcium source if made with calcium chloride or calcium sulfate, I began to realize the potential for tofu in lactose-free cooking.

As I have researched and tested recipes for this book, I have learned to bake without butter, make delectable sauces without cream and use only a whiff of hard cheese for flavor. You do not need to feel deprived if you are lactose intolerant!

Lactose Intolerance Defined

Lactose is the milk sugar found in all animal milk, including human milk. Lactose intolerance is the inability to digest this milk sugar. Most of us are born with lactase, an enzyme found in the digestive tract, which breaks lactose down into two simple sugars: glucose and galactose. If lactase is no longer available to break down lactose into these two simple sugars, the sugar goes on to the large intestine where it becomes fermented by intestinal bacteria. This fermentation causes the symptoms of lactose intolerance—bloating, diarrhea, abdominal pain and gas. Symptoms will vary from individual to individual. With prolonged diarrhea there are the side effects of rectal tenderness, dehydration, weakness and weight loss. Some people will be uncomfortable while, on rare occasions, others will have to be hospitalized.

Primary Intolerance

When lactose intolerance occurs due to the decline in lactase, it is considered primary intolerance. Between the ages of five and seven the activity of this enzyme often declines, and many of the world's adults lose their ability to digest lactose. In fact, most of the world's population cannot digest milk—only Western and Northern Europeans tolerate milk. Many Asians, Hispanics, Mediterraneans, Blacks and Native North Americans are lactose intolerant.

Secondary Intolerance

When lactose intolerance occurs as a result of a disease, this is classed as a secondary intolerance. Some diseases that might result in lactose intolerance are ulcerative colitis, celiac disease, Crohn's disease, viral diarrhea or cancer. In these cases, a reduced-lactose diet is recommended while the symptoms persist and until the system settles down. Once the enzyme begins to work again, regular dairy foods can be reintroduced. If enzyme depletion is permanent, milk containing lactose cannot be reintroduced. Fortunately, there are lactose-reduced milks available as well as tablets that can be taken with milk foods to help digest the lactose. A doctor should be consulted for assistance and a dietitian can help with an appropriate diet.

Milk Allergy

Milk allergy is quite different from lactose intolerance. It is a reaction to the protein in milk, not the sugar, and affects the immune system, causing classic allergy symptoms—wheezing, eczema, rash, mucous build-up, and asthma. Milk allergy usually affects babies or young children and can be serious. The child will be put on a soy formula because to continue with milk will only assault the immune system further. Often the child will outgrow the allergy. Once this happens, milk and milk products can gradually be reintroduced into the diet, but parents should check with the doctor to find out when and if milk can be reintroduced.

Diagnosing Lactose Intolerance

If you suspect you are lactose-intolerant, have your condition checked by your doctor. The doctor may do one of several tests to determine if this is the problem.

Once diagnosed, your doctor or dietitian will put you on a lactose-free diet to clear your system. That means no milk, and no products that contain milk such as whey, curds, cheese, yogurt, sour cream, ice cream, sherbets, butter or margarine containing milk products or cottage cheese.

Each person is affected differently. You may experience discomfort from bloating and diarrhea, but still be able to function. Or you may be quite ill, and it will take longer to return to a healthy balance. You will be put on a plain diet, eating easily digested food such as steamed vegetables and fish with lots of clear fluids. You should get plenty of rest, and cut out caffeine and alcohol. Once your system has calmed down, you can gradually reintroduce small amounts of food that contain lactose.

Finding Your Tolerance Level

As a lactose-intolerant patient, you will receive helpful information from your doctor or dietitian on how to find your tolerance to milk products. It is important to find your tolerance to milk and their products because of their nutrition contribution to your diet.

Every person has a different tolerance level. Some can have yogurt; some cannot. Some can tolerate hard natural cheese (as opposed to soft unripened cheese); some cannot. For some, milk or milk products eaten with a meal in small quantities are easier to digest. It is a trial and error method unique to each individual, and results vary with each individual from time to time.

Start with the most easily digested milk products first and work your way up to find your tolerance level. Remember to go slowly and wait a day in between before including another food. It is reassuring to know that for many lactose-intolerant people the enzyme available in tablet form can help improve their tolerance levels. By taking two or more tablets before eating a food containing lactose, the symptoms are often eliminated or greatly reduced.

Foods in Order of Ease of Digesting for the Lactose Intolerant

1. Plain breads and baked goods
2. Fermented dairy foods like yogurt where the live bacteria helps digest the lactose more easily
3. Aged cheeses with low lactose levels such as aged Cheddar, Gouda, Edam or Parmesan
4. If all goes well, try about 1/4 cup (50 mL) of milk and work up to 1 cup (250 mL) over several days.

Tolerance will also vary according to the level of stress in your life. You may normally tolerate yogurt but if a particular week is difficult, your symptoms may return. You will have to learn to judge.

OBVIOUS SOURCES OF LACTOSE: milk and milk products—chocolate milk, skim, whole, 1% milk, skim milk powder, goat milk products, cottage cheese, ricotta cheese, whipping cream, half and half, yogurt, buttermilk, sour cream, ice cream, ice milk, sherbet, milk puddings

NOT SO OBVIOUS SOURCES OF LACTOSE: cereals produced with skim milk powder, processed meats like sausages and wieners, commercially prepared creamed vegetable dishes like scalloped potatoes or vegetables in a sauce, cream soups, commercial pancakes and waffles, cake mixes, muffin mixes, milk chocolate, chocolate drink mixes, certain prepared cakes, breads, pies and cookies, medications

Lactose is present when the label includes milk, milk solids,
cheese flavor, whey, curds, margarine unless labeled "non-dairy."
Lactose is not present when the ingredient listing includes
lactic acid, lactalbumin, lactate, casein.

You need to know how to read ingredient listings on food labels to know if lactose is present in a particular food—ingredients are listed in order of the greatest quantity to the smallest. Therefore where the ingredient falls in the list will give you some idea of the relative amount in the food.

Small amounts of lactose are added during the processing of numerous foods and drug products. Check with your pharmacist in the case of medications.

The Importance of Milk and Milk Products

Vitamin D

Milk is fortified with Vitamin D, sometimes called the sun vitamin, which prevents us from getting rickets, a disease causing bone deformity and stunted growth. It is essential for the absorption of calcium. Vitamin D is only available in fortified milk (not soy milk), fish oils (cod liver oil and halibut oil) and from exposure to the sun. When the skin is exposed to the sun, it manufactures vitamin D. However, if you are unable to drink milk and have limited access to daily sun or wear sun block, it is a good idea to take a supplement. Check with your doctor or dietitian for the correct amount for your individual needs.

Calcium

Milk and milk products are excellent sources of calcium. In fact, nutrition guidelines often recommend daily servings of milk and milk products from infancy to old age. Obviously, if you are lactose intolerant you may not be able to consume the recommended quantity of milk and will have to incorporate non-dairy sources of calcium into your diet.

WHAT DOES CALCIUM DO FOR US? We need calcium to build strong bones and healthy teeth, for blood clotting, for the proper functioning of muscles, nerves and the heart. You will never outgrow the need for calcium because bone matter is constantly being replaced by new bone.

WE CANNOT PRODUCE CALCIUM OURSELVES. We must eat foods that contain calcium; we then store calcium in our bodies for future use. If we do not eat enough foods containing calcium, our body automatically removes calcium stored in our bones and uses it to carry out the necessary bodily functions.

This constant "borrowing" from our calcium store can lead to a calcium deficiency that is further aggravated by the natural aging process. From about 35 onward, bone loss is likely to be a part of that process. This plus a calcium-deficient diet can result in fragile bones—a condition known as osteoporosis. This is a painful, disabling condition often affecting women after menopause (due to lack of estrogen), and men after the age of 60. It is essential that we have enough calcium in our stores prior to age 35 to combat this process. Once you have been diagnosed by a doctor as lactose intolerant, it will be necessary to find your tolerance level to milk products in order to keep as many as possible in your daily diet, and to make up the difference with the non-dairy sources of calcium (see chart on page 12).

STAGE OF LIFE: You will notice that nutrition recommendations vary depending on your stage of life. For instance, a rapidly growing child, pregnant woman or a nursing mother each has high calcium needs. Again, it is necessary to have enough calcium for this additional growth so that individual stores are not robbed of this mineral.

TO REDUCE RISK OF OSTEOPOROSIS:

- eat calcium-rich foods
- eat a varied diet, making sure you include choices from as many food groups as possible
- perform regular weight-bearing exercise like walking
- drink caffeine and alcohol in moderation

CALCIUM FROM OTHER SOURCES: Fortunately for lactose-intolerant people, milk and milk products are not the only source of calcium. The chart on page 12 lists non-dairy sources of calcium such as almonds, sesame seeds, kale, white beans, broccoli and tofu made with calcium sulfate or calcium chloride. These foods, together with salmon with bones, sardines with bones, lactose-reduced milk, yogurt and aged natural cheeses will be used in this cookbook to boost calcium.

PROTEIN AND CALCIUM ABSORPTION: In many countries where small amounts of protein are eaten and milk is not part of the diet, calcium is better utilized. The more protein ingested, the more calcium is excreted by the body.

BIO-AVAILABILITY AND SOURCES OF CALCIUM: Bio-availability is the amount of the nutrient that can be absorbed and utilized by the body.

For instance, the calcium from milk and milk products has excellent bio-availability—that is, most of the calcium consumed is used by the body. In contrast, there are a number of vegetables like spinach, beet greens, sweet potatoes and rhubarb that are high in calcium but contain oxalic acid, which makes absorption of calcium in the small intestine difficult. Other vegetables from the brassica family are oxalate-free and are a good source of calcium. These are kale, broccoli and bok choy.

Phytates are found in grains and legumes. They too make complete absorption of calcium difficult. Dietary fiber is also associated with reduced calcium absorption.

Surprising Soybeans

There are a number of nutritious foods made from soybeans. They are low in fat, cholesterol free, easily digested, rich in protein and in the case of tofu, when made with calcium sulfate or calcium chloride, a source of calcium. This is not news to people in Asian countries but the foods are relatively new to us in North America (within the last century).

Tofu—What is it?

Tofu, also called soybean curd, is the vegetarian equivalent of cottage cheese in the dairy world. It is made by combining fresh hot soy milk with a coagulant to cause curdling. It is important to note for our purposes that if the coagulant used is calcium sulfate or calcium chloride, tofu becomes a source of calcium. It is also a cholesterol-free source of protein with unsaturated fat. To ensure that you are buying a tofu containing calcium, read the ingredient list on the label for the coagulant. Remember, it must read calcium chloride or calcium sulfate to be a calcium source.

Fat Content of Tofu

Tofu can be high in fat; check the particular type you are using for fat content and use appropriately sized servings. Nevertheless, even though tofu contains fat, it is a lower fat alternative to either sour cream or cream cheese as the nutrient analysis comparison below shows. As you can see, tofu also contributes to protein. When coagulated with calcium choloride or calcium sulfate it becomes a source of calcium too!

COMPARE: ONE SERVING OF	Old-Fashioned Chocolate Cheesecake. made with cream cheese:	Chocolate Cheesecake made with tofu:
Calories	146.8	106.6
Protein	2.5 g	2.3 g
Carbohydrate	16.3 g	16.4 g
Fat	8.4 g	3.4 g
Calcium	20.7 mg	14.2 mg
Dietary Fiber	0.0 g	0.0 g
Percent of carlories from:		
Carbohydrate:	43%	59%
Protein:	7%	8%
Fat:	50%	32%

Not all Tofu is Created Equal

There are two common types of tofu available: cotton and silken.

COTTON TOFU: Soybean milk and the coagulant are combined in a cotton-lined container with holes. Weights are applied to the mixture to firm it up and press out the liquid. Cotton tofu is commonly found at the vegetable counters of supermarkets in soft, firm and extra firm consistencies. Soft tofu is ideal for dressings, sauces and dips; firm tofu is good for cheesecake, puddings and spreads; and extra firm is good for marinating, slicing, grilling and stir frying.

Cotton tofu should be sold from a refrigerated counter like any fragile food. If not, you will not be buying a product at its peak quality. When you get the tofu home, drain the liquid from the tofu and cover it with fresh water. Re-cover and refrigerate. Packages are stamped with an expiry date and must be kept refrigerated; use the tofu by the expiry date listed on the package, changing the water daily.

SILKEN TOFU is made from extra thick soy milk. It is strained through silk, the process giving it the name " silken," but the liquid is not drained off. The result is a creamy custard-like product. As with cotton tofu, soft silken tofu is ideal for dressings, sauces and dips; firm is good for cheesecake, puddings and spreads; and extra firm is good for marinating, slicing, grilling and stir frying.

Silken tofu is vacuum packed and sometimes comes in convenient tetra packs or vacuum packed containers available at health food stores and some grocery stores. It has an expiry date stamped on the package but is shelf stable (if in the tetra pack) for several months; otherwise, refrigerate and use before the expiry date.

Soy Milk

This is the liquid squeezed from soaked soybeans. Soy milk has a beige color and a neutral flavor.

AVAILABILITY: Soy milk can be purchased in the supermarket or health food store, usually aseptically packed with an expiry date on the box. It comes in a variety of flavors—plain, vanilla and chocolate are the most common.

Some stores may have fresh soy milk in a refrigerated section in bottles or cartons. Soy milk also comes powdered in boxes. Once rehydrated, it keeps five days in the refrigerator.

NUTRITION OF SOY MILK

- about the same amount of fat as cow's milk, also available in 1%
- rich in protein
- rich in iron
- contains no calcium (some fortified brands available)
- no vitamin D fortification
- cholesterol free
- low in saturated fat
- lactose-free

Soy milk should not be used for infants. They require the specially prepared commercial soy-based infant formula to fill their nutritional needs.

Tips About Using Tofu and Soy Milk in Recipes

DRAINING TOFU: Tofu needs to be drained in a sieve before adding it to a recipe.

AS A SUBSTITUTE FOR MILK: Tofu and soy milk both have a bland, flat flavor. When we worked with them in the recipes, we found it necessary to add more spices or herbs than we would if we had been using a milk product. If you try to adapt some of your own recipes remember that you cannot substitute soy milk or tofu directly for milk or milk products and expect exactly the same taste results. The soy foods seem to absorb flavorings. However, once additional flavoring is added, the recipe should be tasty.

GARNISH: In the case of soy milk, it may be necessary to add ingredients with more color or add a garnish to compensate for the beige color of the dishes.

ADVANTAGES OF SILKEN TOFU: The convenience of a shelf-stable product and its delicate texture and flavor make it an excellent substitute for sour cream and cream cheese in cheesecake, dips and spreads. Again, added seasoning is required to compensate for the bland taste. Experiment with the different kinds of tofu yourself to see what works best for you.

COOKING: Use extra firm tofu in a recipe to replace meat because it keeps its shape while cooking and has a texture more similar to meat than softer tofu. Because tofu is bland in flavor it is often marinated first before cooking. Like meat, tofu can be browned in hot oil first then cooked on medium or low heat to simmer and absorb the flavors of the dish.

SMOOTH TEXTURE: For a smooth texture use a food processor or blender to purée the soft tofu. This is particularly important in dressings or sauces where a silky consistency is required.

FREEZING TOFU: Leftover tofu can be wrapped carefully and frozen for up to six months. The texture will change but it will make a chewy meat-like substitute for ground meat or crumbled cheese. Defrost the tofu in the refrigerator for 24 hours. Squeeze out the moisture before using.

Do we need milk to get enough calcium?

DEVELOPED BY BRENDA DAVIS, CO-AUTHOR OF *BECOMING VEGETARIAN* (THE BOOK PUBLISHING CO.)

Is it possible to build strong bones without cow's milk? If you grew up in North America you'd probably think not. After all, dairy products are one of the four "essential" food groups and we all know that it's hard to plan a well-balanced diet when a whole food group is left out.

But wait a minute. If dairy foods are so important for good nutrition and more specifically for strong bones, how can it be that the people with the lowest rates of osteoporosis in the world consume little or no dairy at all? It is really quite simple. In addition to positive lifestyle factors such as ample weight-bearing exercise, these people eat plant-centered diets and therefore need less calcium than people who consume a lot of meat. The reason for this is that animal foods tend to be high in sulfur-containing amino acids which cause calcium loss in the urine. Thus in countries where animal foods are a central part of the diet, the recommended daily intake for calcium is set high. For example, the recommended nutrient intake (RNI) for calcium in the United States is approximately 800 mg/day (adults) as compared to 400-500 mg/day suggested by the World Health Organization.

All that having been said, one may still wonder where people who don't use dairy would get their calcium. They generally get it from the same place cows get their calcium—plants. While it is true that dairy products are high in calcium, they are far from being the only good calcium sources. Calcium powerhouses from the plant world include many dark greens, some legumes, nuts and seeds. So, if you have decided to reduce or eliminate dairy from your diet, rest assured that it *is* possible to get enough calcium without milk. The following chart gives a summary of calcium-rich plant foods. Provided in the chart is the following information.

1. Total calcium content per serving. This gives the calcium in mg of calcium per serving. Source: Pennington's Food Values of Portions Commonly Used, 1989.

2. Fractional absorption. This tells us how much calcium we can actually absorb from a food. For example, the figure for broccoli is 53% which means that we can absorb about 53% of the calcium we get from broccoli. The figures were derived from Connie Weaver's work at Purdue University in the United States.

3. Estimated absorbable calcium. This figure tells us how much calcium will be absorbed by our bodies. It is obtained by multiplying the total calcium in a serving of food by its fractional absorption. For example, 1 cup of boiled broccoli has 178 mg of calcium. We multiply 178 by 0.53 (the

fractional absorption) to get the estimated absorbable calcium in broccoli (178 x 0.53 = 94). There is approximately 94 mg of absorbable calcium per cup of boiled broccoli.

Note: If you would like to compare the total calcium in your diet to the Recommended Nutrient Intake (RNI) for calcium (i.e. approximately 800 mg/day in the United States), calculate your intake by using the calcium content of foods column rather than the estimated absorbable calcium column. The reason that we do not use the estimated absorbable calcium figures is that this information is very new and values are not yet available for all foods. In addition, Recommended Nutrient Intakes for calcium are designed to allow for the many factors that affect calcium absorption.

Plant Sources of Calcium

Food	Serving Size	Calcium Content (mg)	Fractional Absorption (%)	Estimated Absorbable Calcium/ Serving (mg)
Almonds, dry roasted	1 oz	80	21	17
Almond butter	1 tbsp	43	21	9
Beans, pinto, red or cranberry	1 cup	82–89	17	14–15
Beans, great northern or navy	1 cup	121–128	17	21–22
Beans, white	1 cup	161	17	27
Blackstrap molasses	1 tbsp	137	n/a	n/a
Broccoli, boiled	1 cup	178	53	94
Brussels sprouts, boiled	1 cup	56	64	36
Cabbage, Chinese, boiled	1 cup	158	54	85
Cabbage, green, boiled	1 cup	50	65	33
Cauliflower, boiled	1 cup	34	69	23
Figs, dried	5 med.	135	n/a	n/a
Kale, boiled	1 cup	94	59	55
Kohlrabi, boiled	1 cup	40	67	27
Mustard greens, boiled	1 cup	104	58	60
Oranges, navel	1 med.	56	n/a	n/a
Rutabaga, boiled	1 cup	72	61	44
Sesame seeds, hulled	1 oz	37	21	8
Sesame seeds, unhulled	1 oz	281	21	58
Sesame seed butter (tahini)	1 tbsp	64	21	13
Soy milk, Semblance	1 cup	200	31	62
Soy milk, Edensoy	1 cup	95	31	29
Soy milk, Vitasoy	1 cup	76	31	24
Spinach, boiled	1 cup	244	51	12
Tofu, set with calcium, firm	1/2 cup	258	31	80
Tofu, set with calcium, medium	1/2 cup	130	31	40
Turnip greens, boiled	1 cup	198	52	103
Milk (for comparison)	1/2 cup	150	32	48

Great Beginnings

Dips, Spreads and Other Nibbles

Your dipping days are not over if you are lactose-intolerant. Typically, appetizers use cream cheese and sour cream as a base. Silken soft and firm tofu can play a major role in replacing these lactose products with excellent results. No one will know the difference!

Tofu tastes bland and absorbs flavors. By adding more herbs and spices than you would when using cream cheese or sour cream, you can compensate for this. Make sure you taste as you are working with the tofu in a recipe and note your preferences of seasonings as you go along. A food processor is a real asset because it can turn tofu into a smooth, creamy dip that would otherwise be lumpy. If a food processor is unavailable, use an electric mixer or blender. These appetizers are easy to digest and are lighter than the original versions because tofu has a lower-fat content than cream cheese or sour cream.

Shelf-stable silken tofu, available from the health food store, has definitely become a staple in my pantry!

Guacamole Spread

Dip tortilla or corn chips into this zesty spread or serve a dollop over sliced tomatoes. It is the perfect companion to chicken salad, whether in a sandwich or in a pita with sprouts. You can keep the spread covered and refrigerated for up to two days.

Makes about 1½ cups
(375 mL)

1	pkg (10.25 oz/290 g) silken soft tofu	1
2 tbsp	fresh lemon juice	25 mL
1 tbsp	vegetable oil	15 mL
2 tsp	Dijon mustard	10 mL
1 tsp	each salt and granulated sugar	5 mL
¼ tsp	black pepper	1 mL
Pinch	cayenne pepper	Pinch
1	ripe avocado, peeled and pitted	1

If an avocado is ripe, it will give slightly to the pressure of your hand without feeling mushy. The skin will be brownish green rather than bright green. If only hard, underripe avocados are available, buy in advance and store in a paper bag or with a bunch of bananas to hasten ripening.

1. Using sieve, drain tofu.

2. In food processor, purée drained tofu, lemon juice, oil, mustard, salt, sugar, black pepper, cayenne pepper and avocado until smooth.

3. Spoon into serving bowl; cover and refrigerate for up to 2 days.

Per serving   (1 tbsp/15 mL)

Calories	23.8
Protein	0.7 g
Carbohydrate	1.1 g
Fat	2.0 g
Calcium	4.9 mg
Dietary Fiber	0.2 g

Percent of calories from:

Carbohydrate:	18%
Protein:	11%
Fat:	71%

Herbed Pâté

Makes about 1⅓ cups
(325 mL)

Silken soft tofu replaces the original recipe's sour cream and cream cheese with less fat, and it provides calcium if made with calcium chloride. Be sure to check the ingredient list on the label for calcium chloride or calcium sulfate. This creamy, garlicky concoction takes minutes to make in a food processor. Serve with a medley of crudités. Be sure to include broccoli and strips of bok choy as a calcium source.

1	pkg (10.25 oz/290 g) silken soft tofu	1
½ cup	chopped fresh parsley	125 mL
2 tbsp	each light mayonnaise, fresh lemon juice and chopped green olives	25 mL
2	green onions, chopped	2
1	clove garlic, minced	1
1 tsp	Worcestershire sauce	5 mL
½ tsp	salt	2 mL
½ tsp	each dried thyme and black pepper	1 mL
Dash	Tabasco sauce	Dash

1. Using sieve, drain tofu.

2. In food processor using pulsing motion or in mixing bowl using electric mixer, combine drained tofu, parsley, mayonnaise, lemon juice, olives, onions, garlic, Worcestershire sauce, salt, thyme, pepper and Tabasco until well blended.

3. Spoon into serving bowl. For best flavor, cover and refrigerate for 1 day. Pâté can be refrigerated for up to 2 days.

Per serving   (1 tbsp/15 mL)

Calories	12.6
Protein	0.7 g
Carbohydrate	0.9 g
Fat	0.8 g
Calcium	7.9 mg
Dietary Fiber	0.1 g

Percent of calories from:

Carbohydrate:	26%
Protein:	22%
Fat:	52%

Double Salmon Spread

Don't forget to include the salmon bones for a calcium boost in this spread. Serve on melba toast garnished with a sprig of dill.

Makes about 1 cup
(250 mL)

1	pkg (10.25 oz/290 g) silken soft tofu	1
1	can (7.5 oz/213 g) sockeye salmon	1
4 oz	smoked salmon	125 g
¼ cup	each dill sprigs and fresh lemon juice	50 mL
2 tbsp	each light mayonnaise and chopped green onion	25 mL
1 tsp	horseradish	5 mL
¼ tsp	black pepper	1 mL

1. Using sieve, drain tofu. Drain sockeye salmon; discard skin and dark pieces, reserving bones.

2. In food processor using pulsing motion, combine drained tofu, salmon with bones, smoked salmon, dill, lemon juice, mayonnaise, onion, horseradish and pepper until smooth.

3. Spoon into serving bowl; cover and refrigerate for up to 2 days.

Per serving   (1 tbsp/15 mL)

Calories	45.0
Protein	4.4 g
Carbohydrate	1.3 g
Fat	2.5 g
Calcium	45.8 mg
Dietary Fiber	0.0 g

Percent of calories from:

Carbohydrate:	11%
Protein:	39%
Fat:	50%

Smoked Salmon Pâté

Makes about 4 cups (1 L)

This elegant pâté, based on the original recipe with oodles of cream, of course, has no cream! It makes a great party appetizer. Garnish with lemon slices and serve with crackers.

This is your chance to use that fancy mold you have been storing. If you don't have one, use a loaf pan lined with plastic wrap instead.

1	pkg (10.25 oz/290 g) silken soft tofu	1
1	package unflavored gelatin	1
¼ cup	water, at room temperature	50 mL
12 oz	smoked salmon	375 g
¼ cup	light mayonnaise	50 mL
2 tbsp	fresh lemon juice	25 mL
¼ tsp	black pepper	1 mL
3	egg whites	3

1. Using sieve, drain tofu.

2. In small saucepan, sprinkle gelatin over water. Set aside.

3. In food processor using pulsing motion, combine drained tofu, salmon, mayonnaise, lemon juice and pepper until smooth.

4. Dissolve gelatin over medium heat about 3 minutes or until clear. With motor running, pour gelatin through feed tube until mixture is well combined.

5. In deep mixing bowl using electric mixer, beat egg whites until standing in stiff peaks. Spoon into salmon mixture. Using on/off pulsing action, combine just until no white shows.

6. Spoon salmon mixture into 4-cup (1 L) mold lined with plastic wrap. Refrigerate for 2 hours until set or overnight.

7. Place serving plate over mold; invert mold and using plastic wrap as a lever, unmold onto plate. Discard plastic wrap. Smooth pâté surface with knife.

Per serving (1 tbsp/15 mL)

Calories	12.2
Protein	1.5 g
Carbohydrate	0.3 g
Fat	0.6 g
Calcium	2.0 mg
Dietary Fiber	0.0 g

Percent of calories from:

Carbohydrate:	9%
Protein:	49%
Fat:	42%

Seafood Pâté

This makes a flavorful sandwich filling or party spread for tortillas. For tortilla spirals, simply spread seafood pâté on tortillas, roll up tightly jelly-roll fashion in plastic wrap, twisting ends and tucking under. Refrigerate until an hour or two before serving, then slice in 2-inch (5 cm) pieces. For best flavor, buy fresh shrimp and cook them for this recipe.

Makes about 4 cups (1 L)

Lemon juice from freshly squeezed lemons gives a flavor superior to bottled concentrate. To get the most juice out of your lemons, let them stand at room temperature to warm up or immerse in hot water for a minute.

1	pkg (10.25 oz/290 g) silken soft tofu	1
2	cans (each 7.5 oz/213 g) sockeye salmon	2
4 oz	cooked fresh shrimp	125 g
¼ cup	light mayonnaise	50 mL
2 tbsp	fresh lemon juice	25 mL
1 tbsp	each ketchup and grated onion	15 mL
1 tsp	Worcestershire sauce	5 mL
Dash	Tabasco sauce	Dash

1. Using sieve, drain tofu. Drain salmon; discard skin and dark pieces, reserving bones.

2. In food processor using pulsing motion, combine drained tofu, salmon with bones, shrimp, mayonnaise, lemon juice, ketchup, onion, Worcestershire sauce and Tabasco until smooth.

3. Spoon into serving bowl; cover and refrigerate for up to 2 days.

Per serving (1 tbsp/15 mL)

Calories	17.1
Protein	1.7 g
Carbohydrate	0.3 g
Fat	1.0 g
Calcium	16.6 mg
Dietary Fiber	0.0 g

Percent of calories from:

Carbohydrate:	8%
Protein:	40%
Fat:	52%

Mexican Tortilla Rolls

Makes about 20 pieces

These colorful sandwiches are popular with all ages. Serve with bowls of salsa, and Tofu Cream (page 50) for dipping.

4	10-inch (25 cm) flour tortillas	4

Leftover tofu can be wrapped and frozen. Although crumbly in texture when defrosted, the tofu can be used in dishes such as chili to replace or supplement meat.

Filling

6 oz	extra firm tofu, crumbled	175 g
¾ cup	salsa	175 mL
½ cup	each sliced black olives and chopped red pepper	125 mL
⅓ cup	chopped fresh coriander	75 mL
2 tbsp	fresh lime juice	25 mL
1 tsp	grated lime rind	5 mL
½ tsp	salt	2 mL
2	green onions, chopped	2

The firmer the tofu, the higher the fat, protein and calcium content.

1. Filling: In food processor using pulsing motion, combine tofu, salsa, olives, red pepper, coriander, lime juice, lime rind, salt and onions.

2. Spread about 1/2 cup (125 mL) filling on each tortilla, leaving 1/2-inch (1 cm) border.

3. Roll up tightly and wrap in plastic wrap. Refrigerate 1 hour or overnight to allow flavors to mellow and to firm up for easy slicing.

4. To serve, unwrap and slice 5 diagonal pieces about 2 inches (10 cm) long. Discard trimmings.

Per serving   (1 piece)

Calories	42.2
Protein	1.3 g
Carbohydrate	5.4 g
Fat	2.0 g
Calcium	27.8 mg
Dietary Fiber	0.6 g

Percent of calories from:

Carbohydrate:	48%
Protein:	12%
Fat:	40%

Mediterranean Crostini

This speedy snack is ideal to serve as a simple appetizer or as an accompaniment to soup or salad for a light meal. Sardines add extra zip and calcium to the topping. Although you can use a commercial tomato sauce for added speed, this flavorful homemade tomato sauce is quick and easy—and too good to miss.

Makes about 35 pieces

1	baguette (16 inches/40 cm long), cut into 1/2-inch (1 cm) thick slices	1
2 cups	Homemade Tomato Sauce (recipe opposite) or commercial thick tomato pasta sauce	500 mL
1	can (100 g) sardines, drained and patted dry	1
1 cup	freshly grated Parmesan cheese (optional, if tolerated)	250 mL

If cheese is not tolerated, crumble firm tofu or defrosted frozen tofu over crostini.

1. Spread each slice of baguette with about 1 tbsp (15 mL) Homemade Tomato Sauce.

2. Coarsely chop sardines; place piece on center of each slice. Sprinkle with cheese, if tolerated. Arrange on baking sheet. Cover and refrigerate for up to 3 hours.

3. Preheat oven to 375°F (190°C). Bake crostini for about 5 minutes or until heated through. Serve immediately.

Homemade Tomato Sauce

2 tbsp	extra virgin olive oil	25 mL
1 cup	finely chopped onions	250 mL
2	cloves garlic, minced	2
1	can (28 oz/796 mL) tomatoes, drained and chopped	1
1	can (5 1/2 oz/156 mL) tomato paste	1
2 tbsp	fresh lemon juice	25 mL
1 tsp	each dried basil and oregano	5 mL
½ tsp	each granulated sugar and salt	2 mL
	Pepper	
¼ cup	chopped fresh parsley	50 mL

1. In saucepan, heat oil over medium-high heat. Add onions and garlic; cook, covered, until onions are softened, about 5 minutes.

2. Stir in tomatoes, tomato paste, lemon juice, basil, oregano, sugar and salt; cook about 5 minutes. Season with pepper to taste. Stir in parsley. Sauce can be covered and refrigerated for up to 1 day. Makes 2 cups (500 mL).

Per serving   (1 piece)

Calories	60.5
Protein	3.2 g
Carbohydrate	7.5 g
Fat	2.8 g
Calcium	70.5 mg
	(a source)
Dietary Fiber	0.7 g

Percent of calories from:

Carbohydrate:	49%
Protein:	21%
Fat:	30%

Spanakopita

These crispy Greek-style triangles are traditionally made with a spinach and cheese mixture, but of course, tofu replaces cheese in this lactose-free version. Kale, similar in taste to spinach but a better calcium source, can be substituted for spinach. (See Braised Kale on page 116 for preparation instructions.) Spanakopita can be made ahead and frozen if desired, to be heated up later and served piping hot.

Makes about 24 pieces

1	pkg (1 lb/500 g) strudel (phyllo) dough	1
⅓ cup	extra virgin olive oil	75 mL

Filling

1	pkg (10.5 oz/290 g) silken firm tofu	1
2 tbsp	olive oil	25 mL
¼ cup	each chopped green onions and onion	50 mL
1	clove garlic, minced	1
2	pkg (each 10 oz/284 g) fresh spinach	2
¼ cup	each chopped fresh dill and parsley	50 mL
2 tbsp	fresh lemon juice	25 mL
1 tsp	salt	5 mL
¼ tsp	black pepper	1 mL
1 cup	soft fresh bread crumbs	250 mL

1. Filling: Using sieve, drain tofu.

2. In large saucepan, heat oil over medium heat; cook green onions, onions and garlic until onions are softened, about 5 minutes. Set aside.

3. Meanwhile, trim and rinse spinach, shaking off excess water. In same saucepan, cook spinach, covered, until wilted. Uncover and continue cooking until moisture has evaporated. Add onion mixture, drained tofu, dill, parsley, lemon juice, salt and pepper; cook a few minutes, stirring to combine. Let cool.

4. Arrange 1 sheet of strudel dough on counter. Using pastry brush, brush lightly with oil. Sprinkle with 1/3 cup (75 mL) bread crumbs. Place second sheet of dough on top. Brush with oil and sprinkle with 1/3 cup (75 mL) bread crumbs. Repeat once; top with sheet of dough to have 4 layers total.

5. Cut each sheet lengthwise into 4 strips. Place 2 tbsp (25 mL) filling at one corner and roll up to make triangle. Repeat with remaining dough and filling to make about 24 pieces.

6. Arrange on baking sheet lined with parchment paper. (May be covered with plastic wrap and foil and frozen up to 1 month.)

7. Preheat oven to 400°F (200°C). Bake 20 to 25 minutes or until golden brown. (Bake frozen in 375°F/190°C oven 25 to 35 minutes.)

Per serving   (1 piece)

Calories	132.6
Protein	4.1 g
Carbohydrate	15.2 g
Fat	6.4 g
Calcium	51.2 mg
Dietary Fiber	1.4 g

Percent of calories from:

Carbohydrate:	45%
Protein:	12%
Fat:	43%

Kale Tart with Sun-Dried Tomatoes and Pine Nuts

Kale, that tangy relative to the cabbage, provides calcium to the diet. It can be found in the vegetable section of the supermarket looking very much like a large version of spinach. Kale tastes similar to spinach, but has a tougher texture that stands up well to boiling and sautéing to be at its delicious best.

Makes 8 servings

1	pkg (10.25 oz/290 g) silken soft tofu	1
1	bunch kale (1 lb/500 g)	1
2 tbsp	extra virgin olive oil	25 mL
2	cloves garlic, minced	2
2	eggs	2
⅓ cup	chopped drained sun-dried tomatoes packed in oil	75 mL
1 tsp	salt	5 mL
¼ tsp	each nutmeg and black pepper	1 mL
¼ cup	toasted pine nuts	50 mL
1 tbsp	grated Parmesan cheese or crumbled extra firm tofu	15 mL

Pastry

1½ cups	all-purpose flour	375 mL
¾ tsp	salt	4 mL
½ cup	shortening	125 mL
¼ cup	cold water	50 mL

1. Using sieve, drain tofu. Preheat oven to 425°F (220°C).

2. Pastry: In mixing bowl, stir together flour and salt. Using pastry blender, cut shortening into flour until in fine crumbs. Stir in water all at once. Form pastry into ball.

3. Roll out pastry between 2 sheets of waxed paper to fit 10-inch (25 cm) pie plate. Remove top layer of waxed paper. Invert pie plate over pastry; invert plate. Discard waxed paper. Gently ease pastry into plate. Flute edges. Cover and refrigerate.

4. In large saucepan, bring about 1 cup (250 mL) water to a boil and cook kale, covered, just until wilted, 4 to 5 minutes. Drain and chop coarsely. In same saucepan, heat oil over medium heat; cook garlic and chopped kale, stirring until tender, about 2 to 3 minutes. Remove from heat. Set aside.

5. In mixing bowl, whisk together drained tofu, eggs, sun-dried tomatoes, salt, nutmeg and pepper. Stir in kale mixture. Spoon into prepared pie shell. Sprinkle evenly with pine nuts and Parmesan cheese.

6. Bake in preheated oven about 20 minutes or until pastry is golden brown. Reduce heat to 350°F (180°C); bake 25 to 30 minutes or until filling is set. Serve warm or at room temperature.

Per serving

Calories	339.2
Protein	9.7 g
Carbohydrate	27.8 g
Fat	21.3 g
Calcium	173.8 mg
	(a high source)
Dietary Fiber	1.4 g

Percent of calories from:

Carbohydrate:	33%
Protein:	11%
Fat:	56%

Salted Almonds

This calcium-bearing nibble is not too heavy to spoil appetites but just right to titillate the palate when served with drinks before dinner. For added spice, try tossing with a little curry powder.

Makes about 3 cups
(750 mL)

1 lb	unblanched almonds	500 g
2 tbsp	vegetable oil	25 mL
1 tsp	salt	5 mL

1. Preheat oven to 350°F (180°C). In mixing bowl, toss almonds with oil until lightly coated.

2. Spread almonds on baking sheet. Bake 12 to 15 minutes or until fragrant and deep golden brown.

3. Return almonds to mixing bowl; toss with salt. Cool. Store in cookie tin up to 1 week or freeze for up to 2 months.

Per serving
1/3 cup/75 mL; 1/10th recipe)

Calories	284.5
Protein	12.3 g
Carbohydrate	8.8 g
Fat	25.2 g
Calcium	177.6 mg
	(a high source)
Dietary Fiber	7.0 g
	(a very high source)

Percent of calories from:

Carbohydrate:	11%
Protein:	16%
Fat:	73%

Pitas Stuffed with Hummus and Sprouts

Makes about 20 pieces

Making these bite-size pockets with sprouts, tahini and white kidney beans enhances the calcium content. Hummus can be made in minutes in the food processor. It's great in a pita pocket but it's yummy with crudités too. Tahini, made from ground sesame seeds, is available in the specialty section of supermarkets and in Middle Eastern food stores.

White kidney beans and sesame seeds are alternate sources of calcium to milk See page 12.

1	can (19 oz/540 mL) white kidney beans, drained	1
4	green onions	4
1	clove garlic, minced	1
½ cup	loosely packed fresh parsley leaves	125 mL
¼ cup	fresh lemon juice	50 mL
2 tbsp	tahini	25 mL
¼ tsp	black pepper	1 mL
20	whole wheat cocktail pitas (about 1 pkg)	20
1½ cups	sunflower or alfalfa sprouts	375 mL

1. In food processor using pulsing action, combine white kidney beans, onions, garlic, parsley, lemon juice, tahini and pepper until mixed.

2. Using sharp knife, cut halfway round seam of pita. Spoon a generous 1 tbsp (15 mL) hummus into pita; top with about 1 tbsp (15 mL) sprouts.

3. Cover and refrigerate up to 8 hours before serving.

Per serving   (1 piece)

Calories	55.4
Protein	2.8 g
Carbohydrate	9.8 g
Fat	0.9 g
Calcium	16.7 mg
Dietary Fiber	2.9 g
	(a source)

Percent of calories from:

Carbohydrate:	66%
Protein:	19%
Fat:	14%

Mushroom Strudel

Serve piping hot with a salad for luncheon or in smaller portions as an appetizer.

Makes 2 strudels, about 14 pieces

| ½ | pkg (1 lb/500 g) strudel (phyllo) dough | ½ |
| ¼ cup | vegetable oil | 50 mL |

Filling

2 tbsp	vegetable oil	25 mL
1	leek, chopped	1
1	clove garlic, minced	1
12 oz	mushrooms, sliced (about 2 cups/500 mL)	375 g
2 tbsp	each fresh lemon juice and dry sherry	25 mL
1 tsp	each dried thyme, Worcestershire sauce and salt	5 mL
½ tsp	each nutmeg and black pepper	2 mL
12 oz	extra firm tofu, crumbled	375 g
2 cups	fresh brown bread crumbs (2 slices)	500 mL
¼ cup	each unblanched almonds and fresh parsley leaves, chopped	50 mL

Remaining phyllo dough can be wrapped in plastic and frozen.

1. Filling: In Dutch oven or saucepan, heat oil over medium heat; cook leek and garlic, covered, about 5 minutes or until leeks are softened.

2. Stir in mushrooms; cook, covered, about 5 minutes or until juices are released.

3. Stir in lemon juice, sherry, thyme, Worcestershire sauce, salt, nutmeg and pepper; cook, uncovered, until liquid is evaporated. Stir in tofu, bread crumbs, almonds and parsley; cook, stirring for 2 minutes.

4. Arrange 1 sheet of strudel dough on counter. Using pastry brush, brush lightly with oil. Place second sheet of dough on top; brush with oil. Repeat once; top with sheet of dough to have 4 layers total. Spread half of the mushroom mixture along long edge of dough. Roll up like jelly roll.

5. Repeat with 4 more sheets of dough and remaining filling.

6. Place on baking sheet lined with parchment paper. Slice strudels almost all the way through on diagonal into 2-inch (5 cm) thick pieces.

7. Preheat oven to 400°F (200°C). Bake for 20 to 25 minutes or until golden brown.

Per serving (1 piece, 1/14th)

Calories	302.9
Protein	6.3 g
Carbohydrate	21.8 g
Fat	9.2 g
Calcium	63.6 mg
	(a source)
Dietary Fiber	1.1 g

Percent of calories from:

Carbohydrate:	28%
Protein:	8%
Fat:	27%

Tex-Mex Bean and Salsa Pyramid Dip

This versatile recipe can be used as an appetizer for a casual party, or as a main-course salad or accompaniment to a barbecue. Use the tortilla chips to scoop up all the delectable mixture. Guacamole Spread (recipe page 16) can replace the tofu mixture for a different taste.

Makes about 10 servings

1	pkg (10.25 oz/290 g) silken soft tofu	1
5 cups	shredded lettuce	1.25 L
1 cup	sunflower or alfalfa sprouts	250 mL
2 tbsp	each light mayonnaise and fresh lemon juice	25 mL
1 cup	salsa	250 mL
1	can (19 oz/540 mL) kidney beans, drained	1
¾ cup	sliced black olives	175 mL
½ cup	chopped sweet red pepper	125 mL
2	green onions, chopped	2
	Tortilla chips	

Check ingredient list on tortilla chips for milk solids before buying.

1. Using sieve, drain tofu.

2. Arrange lettuce and sprouts in single layer on 12-inch (30 cm) round platter.

3. In food processor or mixing bowl with electric mixer, beat together drained tofu, mayonnaise and lemon juice until smooth. Spread on top of lettuce, leaving 1-inch (2.5 cm) border.

4. Spread salsa on top, leaving 1-inch (2.5 cm) border. Sprinkle kidney beans on top of salsa.

5. Pile olives in center. Surround olives with a ring of red pepper. Surround red pepper with ring of onions.

6. Cover with plastic wrap and refrigerate up to 4 hours before serving. Serve with tortilla chips.

Per serving

Calories	144.7
Protein	6.1 g
Carbohydrate	16.1 g
Fat	7.2 g
Calcium	78.8 mg
	(a source)
Dietary Fiber	4.0 g
	(a high source)

Percent of calories from:

Carbohydrate:	42%
Protein:	16%
Fat:	42%

Sun-Dried Tomato and Parsley Pesto Dip

Makes about 2 cups
(500 mL)

Dry-packed sun-dried tomatoes are cheaper than those packed in oil. To rehydrate, cover with boiling water and simmer about 5 minutes. Drain and cover with extra virgin olive oil and minced garlic clove. Refrigerate in a jar for up to 1 week.

Tofu can successfully replace cream cheese in many recipes. To compensate for tofu's bland taste, you may need to use a little more salt, lemon juice and herbs to give the mixture more zip. Tofu, a protein and iron source, is lactose-free and if it is coagulated with calcium sulfate or calcium chloride, it is a calcium source lower in fat than cream cheese.

Serve with sliced baguette and assorted vegetables. Remember to include the calcium carriers such as broccoli and kale! You can substitute 1/2 cup (125 mL) prepared pesto for the homemade.

½ cup	Parsley Pesto	125 mL
8 oz	soft tofu, drained	250 g
6	drained whole sun-dried tomatoes, packed in oil	6
1	clove garlic, minced	1

1. Using sieve, drain tofu.

2. In food processor and using pulsing motion, combine parsley pesto, tofu, tomatoes and garlic; purée until almost smooth.

3. Spoon into serving bowl; cover and refrigerate for up to 2 days.

Parsley Pesto

1 cup	fresh parsley leaves, washed and dried	250 mL
2 tbsp	grated Parmesan cheese (optional, if tolerated)	25 mL
1 tbsp	toasted pine nuts	15 mL
1 tbsp	dried basil	15 mL
1	large clove garlic	1
½ tsp	salt	2 mL
¼ tsp	black pepper	1 mL
¼ cup	extra virgin olive oil	50 mL

1. Parsley Pesto: In food processor, combine parsley, cheese, pine nuts, basil, garlic, salt and pepper until finely chopped. With motor running, pour in oil. Makes 1/2 cup (125 mL).

Per serving   (2 tbsp/25 mL)

Calories	41.2
Protein	2.1 g
Carbohydrate	1.4 g
Fat	3.2 g
Calcium	35.1 mg
Dietary Fiber	0.2 g

Percent of calories from:

Carbohydrate:	18%
Protein:	18%
Fat:	64%

Antojitos

A popular Mexican-style snack, these can be made as hot as you like depending on the peppers used in the recipe. Serve with your favorite salsa or try Salsa (page opposite).

Salsa (page opposite).

Makes about 25 pieces

| 4 | 10-inch (25 cm) flour tortillas | 4 |

Filling

1	pkg (10.5 oz/297 g) silken firm tofu	1
1 tbsp	vegetable oil	15 mL
½ tsp	each salt and granulated sugar	2 mL
¼ cup	each chopped sweet red pepper and jalapeño peppers	50 mL
2 tbsp	chopped black olives	25 mL
	Salsa	

The general rule for peppers is the smaller the pepper the hotter the taste. Jalapeño peppers are small, green cone-shaped peppers much hotter than the large sweet red, green, yellow or orange pepper. They are usually carefully labeled in super-markets but if in doubt, ask!

1. Filling: Using sieve, drain tofu.

2. In food processor, purée drained tofu, oil, salt and sugar until smooth. Stir in red and jalapeño peppers and olives just until combined.

3. Using about 1/3 cup (75 mL) filling for each, spread tortillas to within 1 inch (2.5 cm) of edge. Roll up and wrap tightly in plastic wrap. Refrigerate for up to 4 hours.

4. Preheat oven to 350°F (180°C). Cut antojitos into 1-1/2 inch (4 cm) pieces. Arrange on baking sheet.

5. Bake for about 10 minutes or until heated through. Serve immediately with salsa for dipping.

Per serving

Calories	33.2
Protein	1.2 g
Carbohydrate	3.7 g
Fat	1.5 g
Calcium	15.6 mg
Dietary Fiber	0.3 g

Percent of calories from:

Carbohydrate:	44%
Protein:	15%
Fat:	41%

Salsa

Makes about 2 cups
(500 mL)

This quickly concocted spicy, fresh relish is ideal to make when tomatoes are at their juicy best.

2	tomatoes, chopped	2
Half	sweet green pepper, chopped	Half
¼ cup	chopped green onion	50 mL
2 tbsp	chopped fresh coriander	25 mL
1 tbsp	each chopped jalapeño pepper, lime juice and olive oil	15 mL
2	cloves garlic, minced	2
1 tsp	red wine vinegar	5 mL
½ tsp	salt	2 mL
Pinch	black pepper	Pinch

1. In mixing bowl, stir together tomatoes, green pepper, green onion, coriander, jalapeño pepper, lime juice, oil, garlic, red wine vinegar, salt and pepper.

2. Serve immediately or cover and let stand at room temperature for up to 2 hours.

Per serving   (1 tbsp/15 mL)

Calories	5.8
Protein	0.1 g
Carbohydrate	0.5 g
Fat	0.4 g
Calcium	2.1 mg
Dietary Fiber	0.1 g

Percent of calories from:

Carbohydrate:	30%
Protein:	6%
Fat:	64%

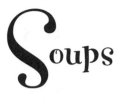

Soups

THERE IS a soup to please every palate and every lifestyle. In addition to your favorite soups such as vegetable, chunky meat or bean, you can still continue to enjoy cream soups and chowders that normally use milk, cream and butter. Vegetable oil, olive oil or a little water replaces butter to sauté vegetables. A vegetable purée thickens soup, giving it a smooth consistency with no lactose. When soups need to be thinned, use stock, lactose-reduced milk, soy milk or even fruit juice to create the desired consistency.

With vegetable purées and a minimum of vegetable oil for cooking, these soups have a lower fat level than the traditional recipes.

Happily, soups can fill the role of lunch or a simple supper when accompanied with good bread and a salad. Soups can be made ahead and in most cases frozen for up to two months. Simply pour it into a plastic container such as a yogurt or margarine tub, label, and freeze. They can be reheated directly from the frozen state, making them ideal to tote along for a work lunch, providing a microwave oven or stove is available. If not, simply reheat and fill a Thermos.

Whole Wheat Croutons

Commercial croutons can be a hidden source of lactose—either in the bread or seasoning. Check the label for skim milk powder or milk solids. Better yet, make your own to be on the safe side, such as these "too good to be true" croutons. Beware, they taste so good for nibbling, there may not be any left for the soup.

Makes about 1⅔ cups (400 mL)

2 tbsp	extra virgin olive oil	25 mL
1	clove garlic, minced	1
4	slices whole wheat day-old bread	4

1. Preheat oven to 375°F (190°C).

2. In small bowl, combine oil and garlic.

3. Using pastry brush, paint over lightly both sides of bread.

4. Trim crusts and cut bread into 1/2-inch (1 cm) cubes. Bake on baking sheets for 20 to 25 minutes or until golden brown.

Per serving
(1/3 cup/75 mL; 1/5th recipe)

Calories	95.8
Protein	2.1 g
Carbohydrate	11.4 g
Fat	5.2 g
Calcium	20.1 mg
Dietary Fiber	1.3 g

Percent of calories from:

Carbohydrate:	45%
Protein:	8%
Fat:	46%

Sweet Potato Orange Soup

Makes about 8 cups (2 L)

Rich and oh-so-smooth, this soup is creamy without cream! Serve with homemade Whole Wheat Croutons (recipe opposite).

Commercial stocks tend to be saltier than homemade stocks. Taste before adding salt.

2 lb	sweet potatoes, peeled and sliced (about 3 large)	1 kg
2 cups	chicken stock	500 mL
2 cups	orange juice	500 mL
1 cup	water	250 mL
1	onion, chopped	1
1	bay leaf	1
1 tsp	dried thyme	5 mL
½ cup	soy milk or 2% lactose-reduced milk	125 mL
½ tsp	salt	2 mL
¼ tsp	black pepper	1 mL

1. In large saucepan, combine potatoes, chicken stock, orange juice, water, onion, bay leaf and thyme. Bring to boil; reduce heat and simmer, covered, for 25 to 30 minutes or until potatoes are very tender. Discard bay leaf.

2. In blender or food processor, process potato mixture, in batches, until smooth. Add milk, salt and pepper; blend well. Gently reheat if necessary to serve.

3. Soup can be refrigerated in airtight container for up to 3 days. Or freeze in individual servings or large container for up to 2 months.

Per serving (1 cup/250 mL)

Calories	137.8
Protein	3.7 g
Carbohydrate	29.6 g
Fat	0.8 g
Calcium	40.6 mg
Dietary Fiber	3.8 g
	(a source)

Percent of calories from:

Carbohydrate:	84%
Protein:	11%
Fat:	5%

Creamy Carrot Soup

Serve this piping hot on a fresh fall day or chilled on a warm summer's day with a dollop of yogurt, if tolerated.

Makes about 8 cups (2 L)

2 tbsp	vegetable oil	25 mL
6	large carrots, peeled and chopped (about 2 lb/1 kg)	6
1	onion, chopped	1
¼ cup	all-purpose flour	50 mL
6 cups	chicken stock	1.5 L
1	bay leaf	1
½ tsp	each salt and dried thyme	2 mL
¼ tsp	black pepper	1 mL
¼ cup	chopped fresh coriander or parsley	50 mL

For a creamy texture, a blender works better for puréeing soup than a food processor.

1. In large saucepan, heat oil; cook carrots and onion over low heat, covered, until carrots are tender, 15 to 20 minutes.

2. Sprinkle with flour; cook, stirring, until flour is pale brown.

3. Gradually whisk in chicken stock, bay leaf, salt, thyme and pepper. Bring to boil; reduce heat and simmer until thickened, about 20 minutes. Discard bay leaf.

4. In blender or food processor, purée soup in batches until smooth. Taste and add more salt if necessary. Serve garnished with coriander.

5. Refrigerate in airtight container for up to 2 days. Or freeze in individual servings or large container for up to 2 months.

Per serving   (1 cup/250 mL)

Calories	120.4
Protein	5.4 g
Carbohydrate	15.8 g
Fat	4.2 g
Calcium	44.9 mg
Dietary Fiber	3.1 g
	(a source)

Percent of calories from:

Carbohydrate:	52%
Protein:	18%
Fat:	31%

Leek and Potato Soup

Makes about 8 cups (2 L)

A hearty soup for a blustery day, this has traditionally been made with cream. This version gives the same rich sensation but with no dairy product!

Leeks are grown in sand. As a result, you need to wash them thoroughly so the sand doesn't end up in the soup! Trim the root end and cut the leek to use only the white and pale green parts. The rest is too coarse, so discard. Slice it lengthwise and rinse under cold running water to penetrate all the crevices and remove any sand.

2 tbsp	vegetable oil	25 mL
2	leeks (white part only), cleaned and sliced	2
4	potatoes, peeled and diced (1¼ lb/625 g)	4
4 cups	chicken stock	1 L
1	bay leaf	1
½ tsp	each dried thyme and black pepper	2 mL
	Salt to taste	
	Whole Wheat Croutons (page 38) or 2 green onions, chopped	

To minimize fat content, add a little water instead of more oil to help vegetables soften without scorching.

1. In large saucepan, heat oil over medium heat; cook leeks, covered, for about 5 minutes or until softened.

2. Add potatoes, chicken stock, bay leaf, thyme and pepper. Cover. Bring to boil; reduce heat and simmer for about 20 minutes or until potatoes are very tender. Discard bay leaf. Taste and add salt if necessary. Serve garnished with croutons.

3. Soup can be refrigerated in airtight container for up to 2 days.

Per serving (1 cup/250 mL)

Calories	125.1
Protein	4.2 g
Carbohydrate	19.1 g
Fat	3.8 g
Calcium	32.3 mg
Dietary Fiber	2.0 g
	(a source)

Percent of calories from:

Carbohydrate:	60%
Protein:	13%
Fat:	27%

Creamy Pumpkin and Apple Soup

Truly a harvest blend made from pumpkin and apple, this soup is puréed and has a velvety texture. For a calcium boost, serve with a spoonful of yogurt, if tolerated, or Yogurt Substitute (page 45).

Makes about 6 cups
(1.5 L)

2 tbsp	vegetable oil	25 mL
2	stalks celery, sliced (1 cup/250 mL)	2
1	large onion, chopped	1
1	can (14 oz/398 mL) pumpkin purée	1
1	apple, peeled, cored and quartered	1
3 cups	chicken stock	750 mL
1	bay leaf	1
1 tsp	curry powder	5 L
¼ tsp	black pepper	1 mL
	Salt to taste	

1. In large saucepan, heat oil over medium heat; cook celery and onion, covered, for about 5 minutes or until softened.

2. Stir in pumpkin, apple, chicken stock, bay leaf and curry powder. Bring to boil; reduce heat and simmer, covered, about 20 minutes or until vegetables are tender. Discard bay leaf.

3. In blender or food processor, purée soup, in batches, until smooth. Stir in pepper and salt to taste.

4. Soup can be refrigerated in airtight container for up to 2 days. Or freeze in individual servings or large container for up to 2 months.

Per serving (1 cup/250 mL)

Calories	101.2
Protein	3.7 g
Carbohydrate	11.9 g
Fat	4.9 g
Calcium	43.4 mg
Dietary Fiber	2.7 g
	(a high source)

Percent of calories from:

Carbohydrate:	45%
Protein:	14%
Fat:	41%

*C*ream of Butternut Squash Soup

Makes about 6 cups (1.5 L)

A vibrant harvest soup, this is perfect served with a spoonful of yogurt, if tolerated, or Yogurt Substitute (page 45) and a grating of fresh nutmeg. Make the most of packaged frozen butternut squash to save time!

2 tbsp	vegetable oil	25 mL
1	onion, chopped	1
1	clove garlic, minced	1
4 cups	cubed peeled squash (fresh or frozen)	1 L
3 cups	chicken stock	750 mL
1	bay leaf	1
½ cup	soy milk or 2% lactose-reduced milk	125 mL
½ tsp	each salt and nutmeg	2 mL
¼ tsp	black pepper	1 mL

1. In large saucepan, heat oil over medium heat; cook onion and garlic, covered, until onions are softened, about 5 minutes.

2. Add squash, chicken stock and bay leaf. Bring to boil; reduce heat and simmer, covered, for 20 to 30 minutes or until squash is very tender. Discard bay leaf.

3. In blender or food processor, purée soup, in batches, until smooth. Stir in milk, salt, nutmeg and pepper. Taste and add more salt if necessary.

4. Soups can be refrigerated in airtight container for up to 2 days. Or freeze in individual servings or large container for up to 2 months.

Per serving (1 cup/250 mL)

Calories	123.4
Protein	4.5 g
Carbohydrate	17.0 g
Fat	5.2 g
Calcium	68.6 mg
	(a source)
Dietary Fiber	3.5 g
	(a source)

Percent of calories from:

Carbohydrate:	51%
Protein:	14%
Fat:	35%

Curried Parsnip Soup

Served hot or cold, this soup has a nutty, sweet flavor complemented by a crunchy calcium topping of toasted almonds.

Makes about 8 cups (2 L)

2 lb	parsnips, peeled and chopped	1 kg
1	onion, chopped	1
1	pear, peeled, cored and quartered	1
1	bay leaf	1
1 tsp	curry powder	5 mL
5 cups	chicken stock	1.25 L
¼ cup	unblanched almonds, chopped	50 mL
1 cup	soy milk or 2% lactose-reduced milk	250 mL
½ tsp	salt	2 mL
¼ tsp	black pepper	1 mL

Toasting nuts or sesame seeds intensifies their flavor. To toast almonds, bake in preheated 350°F (180°C) oven about 15 minutes or until golden brown.

1. In large saucepan, combine parsnips, onion, pear, bay leaf, curry powder and chicken stock. Bring to boil; reduce heat and simmer, covered, for 25 to 30 minutes or until parsnips are very tender. Discard bay leaf.

2. Meanwhile, preheat oven to 350°F (180°C); toast almonds on baking sheet for about 15 minutes or until fragrant and golden brown.

3. In blender or food processor, purée soup, in batches, until smooth. Stir in milk, salt and pepper. Reheat gently in saucepan. Serve garnished with almonds.

4. Soup can be refrigerated in airtight container for up to 2 days. Or freeze in individual servings or large container for up to 2 months.

Per serving (1 cup/250 mL)

Calories	169.8
Protein	6.7 g
Carbohydrate	30.0 g
Fat	3.6 g
Calcium	72.7 mg
	(a source)
Dietary Fiber	7.8 g
	(a very high source)

Percent of calories from:

Carbohydrate:	67%
Protein:	15%
Fat:	18%

Broccoli Tarragon Soup

Makes about 5 cups
(1.2 L)

Broccoli is a vegetable source of calcium. As well, the calcium content of the soup can be enriched if garnished with a spoonful of yogurt, providing yogurt is tolerated. Otherwise, serve with Yogurt Substitute or Sour Cream Substitute (this page).

Yogurt Substitute:
In small bowl, stir together 1 cup (250 mL) drained silken soft tofu with 1 tbsp (15 mL) each vegetable oil and lemon juice until smooth. Makes about 1 cup (250 mL).

Sour Cream Substitute:
In small bowl, stir together 1 cup (250 mL) drained soft tofu with 1 tbsp (15 mL) each light mayonnaise and lemon juice until smooth. Makes about 1 cup (250 mL).

1	bunch broccoli	1
1	onion, chopped	1
1	potato, peeled and chopped	1
1	bay leaf	1
3 cups	chicken stock	750 mL
1 tbsp	dried tarragon	15 mL
	Salt and pepper	
¼ cup	plain yogurt	50 mL

1. Trim tough parts of broccoli stem. Coarsely chop broccoli.

2. In large saucepan, combine broccoli, onion, potato, bay leaf, chicken stock and tarragon. Bring to boil; reduce heat and simmer, covered, until vegetables are tender, 20 to 25 minutes. Discard bay leaf.

3. In blender or food processor, purée soup, in batches, until smooth. Season to taste with salt and pepper. Serve garnished with dollop of yogurt.

4. Soup can be refrigerated in airtight container for up to 2 days. Or freeze in individual servings or large container for up to 2 months.

Per serving (1 cup/250 mL)

Calories	104.5
Protein	7.5 g
Carbohydrate	17.5 g
Fat	1.3 g
Calcium	88.3 mg
	(a source)
Dietary Fiber	3.1 g
	(a source)

Percent of calories from:

Carbohydrate:	63%
Protein:	27%
Fat:	11%

Mushroom Chowder

Serve steaming bowls of this chowder with Whole Grain Seed and Nut Bread (page 132) and a salad for lunch or supper. Don't be afraid to experiment with the various mushrooms available in the supermarket. In fact, brown mushrooms such as cremini mushrooms give this a rich, mellow flavor.

Makes 6 cups (1.5 L)

2	slices bacon, diced	2
1	onion, chopped	1
1	stalk celery, diced	1
1	clove garlic, minced	1
2 cups	sliced mushrooms (½ lb/250 g)	500 mL
2 tsp	dried tarragon	10 mL
1 tbsp	all-purpose flour	15 mL
4 cups	chicken stock	1 L
2	large potatoes, peeled and diced (about 2 ½ cups/625 mL)	2
½ cup	dry white wine	125 mL
½ tsp	each salt and black pepper	2 mL
¼ cup	chopped fresh parsley	50 mL

1. In large saucepan over medium-low heat, cook bacon, onion, celery, garlic, mushrooms and tarragon, covered, until onions are tender and mushrooms release liquid, 5 to 8 minutes.

2. Sprinkle with flour and stir in. Gradually whisk in chicken stock, stirring, until thickened and smooth.

3. Add potatoes, wine, salt and pepper. Increase heat to medium; cook for about 20 minutes or until potatoes are tender.

4. Soup can be prepared to this point and refrigerated in airtight container for up to 2 days; reheat gently. Do not freeze. To serve, stir in parsley.

Per serving (1 cup/250 mL)

Calories	147.2
Protein	7.4 g
Carbohydrate	21.1 g
Fat	3.0 g
Calcium	43.9 mg
Dietary Fiber	2.4 g
	(a source)

Percent of calories from:

Carbohydrate:	55%
Protein:	19%
Fat:	17%

Salmon Chowder

Makes 8 cups (2 L)

Sockeye salmon gives this chowder a lovely pink tinge but any salmon will do. Remember to include the calcium-rich bones. Serve with Whole Grain Seed and Nut Bread (page 132).

2 tbsp	vegetable oil	25 mL
1	onion, chopped	1
1	stalk celery, diced	1
1	carrot, peeled and diced	1
1	clove garlic, minced	1
4 cups	chicken stock	1 L
2	potatoes, peeled and diced	2
1	can (7.5 oz/213 g) sockeye salmon	1
1 cup	dry white wine	250 mL
¼ cup	chopped fresh dill	50 mL
	Black pepper to taste	

1. In large saucepan, heat oil over medium heat; cook onion, celery, carrot and garlic for 8 to 10 minutes or until softened but not browned.

2. Stir in chicken stock and potatoes. Bring to boil; reduce heat and simmer, covered, for about 20 minutes or until potatoes are tender.

3. Drain salmon; discard skin, reserving bones. Add salmon and crushed bones, wine and dill to soup. Return to boil. Season to taste with pepper.

4. Soup can be refrigerated in airtight container for up to 2 days. Do not freeze.

Per serving (1 cup/250 mL)

Calories	157.9
Protein	8.2 g
Carbohydrate	11.8 g
Fat	6.4 g
Calcium	105.9 mg
	(a source)
Dietary Fiber	1.4 g

Percent of calories from:

Carbohydrate:	30%
Protein:	21%
Fat:	37%

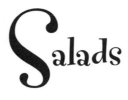alads

SALAD DRESSINGS frequently use sour cream, buttermilk or sometimes cream cheese to give that luscious, rich texture and flavor. Again, silken soft tofu replaces these ingredients and along with added herbs and seasonings it makes luxuriant sauces. You will find a food processor is a real asset to whipping up the dressings and creating the smooth texture.

These lactose-free salads incorporate tofu made with calcium chloride or calcium sulfate, vegetables containing calcium (see chart page 12), additional herbs, and toasted nuts or seeds for taste, texture and added calcium.

Tofu Cream

Tofu makes a lower-fat, calcium-enriched, mayonnaise-like dressing. It works well as a spread or base for other creamy dressings like ranch and Thousand Island.

Makes about 1 cup
(250 mL)

1	pkg (10.25 oz/290 g) silken soft tofu	1
2 tbsp	fresh lemon juice	25 mL
1 tbsp	vegetable oil	15 mL
2 tsp	Dijon mustard	10 mL
1 tsp	each salt and granulated sugar	5 mL
¼ tsp	black pepper	1 mL
Pinch	cayenne pepper	Pinch

1. Using sieve, drain tofu.

2. In food processor using pulsing motion, combine drained tofu, lemon juice, oil, mustard, salt, sugar, pepper and cayenne; purée until smooth.

3. Cream can be refrigerated in airtight container for up to 2 days.

Per serving   (1 tbsp/15 mL)

Calories	19.6
Protein	0.9 g
Carbohydrate	0.9 g
Fat	1.4 g
Calcium	6.5 mg
Dietary Fiber	0.0 g

Percent of calories from:

Carbohydrate:	18%
Protein:	18%
Fat:	64%

Caesar Salad with Creamy Garlic Dressing

Makes 4 servings

The creamy dressing makes a great dip for calcium-containing veggies, too, such as small kale leaves or broccoli florets.

Per serving

Salad with dressing:

Calories	572.1
Protein	36.9 g
Carbohydrate	23.2 g
Fat	37.7 g
Calcium	821.1 mg
Dietary Fiber	3.9 g

Percent of calories from:

Carbohydrate:	22%
Protein:	26%
Fat:	52%

Per serving   (2 tbsp/25 mL)

Dressing:

Calories	39.8
Protein	1.8 g
Carbohydrate	2.0 g
Fat	2.8 g
Calcium	13.7 mg
Dietary Fiber	0.0 g

Percent of calories from:

Carbohydrate:	19%
Protein:	18%
Fat:	63%

Probably the most popular salad on any menu, this version has plenty of zing with just a hint of cheese for flavor. If your tolerance to fresh Parmesan is low, substitute more croutons, a sprinkling of chopped sardines or chopped Salted Almonds (page 28).

1	head, romaine lettuce	1
1	recipe Whole Wheat Croutons (page 38)	1
1 cup	freshly grated Parmesan cheese (optional, if tolerated)	250 mL
½ cup	chopped sardines or chopped sun-dried tomatoes	125 mL

Creamy Garlic Dressing

1	pkg (10.25 oz/290 g) silken soft tofu	1
1	clove garlic, minced	1
2 tbsp	fresh lemon juice	25 mL
1 tbsp	vegetable oil	15 mL
2 tsp	Dijon mustard	10 mL
1 tsp	each salt and granulated sugar	5 mL
¼ tsp	black pepper	1 mL
Pinch	cayenne pepper	Pinch

1. Using sieve, drain tofu.

2. Tear lettuce into bite-size pieces. Cover and refrigerate until ready to toss. May be assembled 1 day ahead of serving. Sprinkle with croutons, cheese (if using) and sardines.

3. Creamy Garlic Dressing: In food processor, purée tofu, garlic, lemon juice, oil, mustard, salt, sugar, pepper and cayenne. Dressing can be refrigerated in airtight container for up to 2 days.

4. Pour dressing over salad; toss to coat evenly.

Nice 'N' Nutty Slaw

Instead of the usual creamy coleslaw dressing, this oil-and-vinegar version allows you to marinate the slaw for several days. Calcium is boosted with the crunch of sesame seeds, sprouts and almonds. Feel free to experiment with your own combination of shredded vegetables; try including some of those containing calcium (see page 12).

Makes 8 servings

½ cup	sliced unblanched almonds	125 mL
¼ cup	sesame seeds	50 mL
3 cups	each shredded red and green cabbage	750 mL
2 cups	sunflower sprouts or alfalfa sprouts	500 mL
1 cup	sliced fennel or celery	250 mL
3	green onions, sliced	3
½ cup	chopped fresh parsley	125 mL
1	apple, cored and sliced	1

Poppyseed Dressing

¼ cup	white wine vinegar or fresh lemon juice	50 mL
2 tbsp	chopped onion	25 mL
2 tbsp	granulated sugar	25 mL
1 tbsp	poppyseeds	15 mL
½ tsp	salt	2 mL
¼ tsp	black pepper	1 mL
¼ cup	vegetable oil	50 mL

1. Preheat oven to 350°F (180°C). Spread almonds and sesame seeds on baking sheet. Bake for 10 to 12 minutes or until golden brown. Let cool.

Fennel is a slightly sweet, licorice-flavored vegetable with the crunch of celery. If you have difficulty finding it in your local supermarket, look in your Italian fruit and vegetable store.

2. In large bowl, combine red and green cabbage, sprouts, fennel, green onions and parsley. Salad can be prepared to this point, covered and refrigerated for up to 1 day.

3. Poppyseed Dressing: In small bowl, whisk together vinegar, onion, sugar, poppyseeds, salt and pepper. Whisk in oil. Dressing can be covered and refrigerated for up to 2 weeks.

4. Up to 4 hours before serving, toss almonds, sesame seeds and apples with cabbage mixture; toss with dressing until well mixed. (Longer marinating will cause apples to brown and almonds to become soggy.)

Per serving

Calories	117.7
Protein	4.6 g
Carbohydrate	13.0 g
Fat	6.8 g
Calcium	145.5 mg
	(a source)
Dietary Fiber	5.0 g
	(a high source)

Percent of calories from:

Carbohydrate:	40%
Protein:	14%
Fat:	46%

Spinach, Almond and Orange Salad

With Creamy Tarragon Dressing

This is a perfect accompaniment to chicken or fish dishes.

½ cup	chopped unblanched almonds	125 mL
1	pkg (10 oz/284 g) fresh spinach	1
2	seedless navel oranges	2
Quarter	red onion, thinly sliced	Quarter

Creamy Tarragon Dressing

1	pkg (10.25 oz/290 g) silken soft tofu	1
2 tbsp	light mayonnaise	25 mL
1 tbsp	white wine vinegar	15 mL
2 tsp	each dried tarragon and granulated sugar	10 mL
1 tsp	each Dijon mustard and salt	5 mL
¼ tsp	black pepper	1 mL

1. Preheat oven to 350°F (180°C). Bake almonds on baking sheet for 10 to 12 minutes or until golden brown. Let cool.

2. Trim spinach; tear into bite-size pieces. Using sharp knife, cut away peel and white pith from oranges; slice crosswise into thin circles.

3. In large salad bowl, combine spinach, orange slices and onion. Cover and refrigerate until ready to toss with dressing. May be assembled for up to 4 hours ahead.

4. Creamy Tarragon Dressing: Using sieve, drain tofu. In blender or food processor using pulsing motion, combine drained tofu, mayonnaise, vinegar, tarragon, sugar, mustard, salt and pepper until smooth. Pour into jar and refrigerate for up to 2 days. Makes enough dressing for 2 salads.

5. Just before serving, toss salad with about 1/2 the dressing or enough dressing to coat.

Makes 6 servings

Per serving

Salad with dressing:

Calories	123.9
Protein	5.8 g
Carbohydrate	15.2 g
Fat	5.9 g
Calcium	124.2 mg
	(a source)
Dietary Fiber	4.1 g
	(a high source)

Percent of calories from:

Carbohydrate:	45%
Protein:	17%
Fat:	39%

Per serving   (1 tbsp/15 mL)

Dressing:

Calories	46.5
Protein	2.5 g
Carbohydrate	3.8 g
Fat	2.5 g
Calcium	22.8 mg
Dietary Fiber	0.0 g

Percent of calories from:

Carbohydrate:	32%
Protein:	21%
Fat:	47%

French Potato Salad

Makes 8 servings

An early summer treat, this tastes wonderful using the tiny garden-fresh new potatoes. Instead of the usual creamy mayo-dressed potato salad, try this tangy marinade that's free of dairy—making it safe to tote on picnics.

| 2 lb | tiny new potatoes or quartered larger potatoes (8 cups/2 L) | 1 kg |

Marinade

½ cup	vegetable oil	125 mL
¼ cup	each white wine vinegar and white wine	50 mL
1 tsp	each Dijon mustard, salt and dried tarragon	5 mL
¼ tsp	black pepper	1 mL
2 tbsp	each chopped fresh parsley and chives	25 mL

1. Scrub but do not peel potatoes. Steam until tender, 15 to 20 minutes. Transfer to bowl.

2. Marinade: In small bowl, whisk together oil, vinegar, wine, mustard, salt, tarragon and pepper. Pour over warm potatoes.

3. Sprinkle potatoes with parsley and chives; toss gently. Serve at room temperature. Salad can be covered and refrigerated for up to 2 days.

Per serving

Calories	243.1
Protein	2.5 g
Carbohydrate	25.8 g
Fat	14.6 g
Calcium	13.3 mg
Dietary Fiber	2.0 g
	(a source)

Percent of calories from:

Carbohydrate:	42%
Protein:	4%
Fat:	53%

Salmon and Wild Rice Salad

Try this salad throughout the seasons, varying the vegetables with the freshest ones available. Use the salmon bones for added calcium. When you accompany this with good bread like Whole Grain Seed and Nut Bread (page 132) or Double Cornbread (page 134), and a green salad in spring or summer or hearty soup in fall or winter, you have a satisfying meal.

Makes 6 servings

1 cup	wild rice	250 mL
1½ tsp	salt	7 mL
2	bay leaves	2
1 cup	long grain parboiled rice	250 mL
1 lb	broccoli florets	500 g
2	cans (each 7.5 oz/213 g) sockeye salmon	2
2 cups	whole button mushrooms (8 oz/250 g)	500 mL
½ cup	chopped fresh parsley	125 mL
4	green onions, chopped	4
Half	sweet red pepper, chopped	Half

Dressing

½ cup	vegetable oil	125 mL
¼ cup	red wine vinegar	50 mL
1 tbsp	granulated sugar	15 mL
1	clove garlic, minced	1
½ tsp	salt	2 mL
¼ tsp	black pepper	1 mL

Peas, asparagus spears, green beans, fiddleheads or sliced zucchini may be substituted for broccoli florets.

To prepare asparagus, break off tough root end. Slice zucchini; leave green beans whole but cut off ends. Fiddleheads are the tightly coiled fronds of the ostrich fern. They need to be rinsed in several changes of water to remove any debris. Trim root end. All green vegetables should be cooked uncovered to maintain their bright green color.

1. Rinse wild rice and cover with cold water. Let soak 30 minutes. Drain.

2. In saucepan, bring 3 cups (750 mL) water, 1 tsp (5 mL) of the salt and 1 of the bay leaves to boil. Stir in wild rice; bring back to boil. Reduce heat and cook, covered, until tender, about 25 minutes. Drain and cool. Discard bay leaf.

3. In separate saucepan, bring 2 cups (500 mL) water, remaining salt and bay leaf to boil. Add parboiled rice; simmer, covered, 15 minutes. Remove from heat and let stand, covered, another 5 minutes or until all liquid is absorbed. Cool. Discard bay leaf.

4. Meanwhile, in saucepan of rapidly boiling salted water, cook uncovered broccoli until tender-crisp, 2 to 3 minutes. Drain and refresh under cold water.

5. Drain salmon; discard skin, reserving bones. In mixing bowl, combine cooled wild and parboiled rice, broccoli, mushrooms, parsley, green onions, red pepper and salmon with crushed bones.

6. Dressing: In small bowl, whisk together oil, vinegar, sugar, garlic, salt and pepper. Pour over salad and toss gently. Salad can be covered and refrigerated for up to 1 day.

Per serving

Calories	550.0
Protein	21.8 g
Carbohydrate	55.7 g
Fat	27.9 g
Calcium	232.4 mg
	(a high source)
Dietary Fiber	2.6 g
	(a source)

Percent of calories from:

Carbohydrate:	40%
Protein:	16%
Fat:	45%

Layered Salad with Ranch-Style Dressing

This is truly a salad for all seasons because you can change the ingredients with the changing crops. It's a great salad for taking to potlucks or picnics, because it can be assembled ahead and tossed at the last minute. By including almonds and beans, you have a source of calcium, fiber and protein.

1	pkg (10 oz/284 g) fresh spinach, or head romaine, washed and dried	1
2 cups	sliced mushrooms (8 oz/250 g)	500 mL
1	red onion, thinly sliced	1
1	can (19 oz/284 mL) white or red kidney beans, drained	1
1	sweet red pepper, chopped	1
2	stalks celery, sliced	2
½ cup	toasted unblanched almonds, chopped coarsely	125 mL

Ranch-Style Dressing

1	pkg (10.25 oz/290 g) silken soft tofu	1
2 tbsp	each light mayonnaise and white wine vinegar	25 mL
1 tbsp	granulated sugar	15 mL
1	clove garlic, crushed	1
1 tsp	salt	5 mL
¼ tsp	black pepper	1 mL

Makes 8 servings

Toasting almonds intensifies the nutty flavor. To toast nuts, arrange in single layer on baking sheet and bake in preheated oven at 350°F (180°C) for 10 to 15 minutes or until fragrant.

Per serving

Salad:

Calories	130.3
Protein	7.8 g
Carbohydrate	15.0 g
Fat	5.9 g
Calcium	97.8 mg
	(a source)
Dietary Fiber	5.0 g
	(a high source)

Percent of calories from:

Carbohydrate:	42%
Protein:	22%
Fat:	37%

1. Ranch-Style Dressing: Using sieve, drain tofu.

2. Meanwhile, tear spinach into bite-size pieces; arrange half over bottom of 9-inch (225 cm) salad bowl. Sprinkle evenly with half of mushrooms, red onion, beans, red pepper and celery. Layer remaining ingredients on top.

3. In food processor using pulsing motion, purée tofu, mayonnaise, vinegar, sugar, garlic, salt and pepper until smooth.

4. Spread dressing over top of spinach layer. Sprinkle with almonds. Cover and refrigerate for up to 1 day. To serve, spoon through layers so that each serving contains all ingredients.

Per serving   (1 tbsp/15 mL)

Dressing:

Calories	35.6
Protein	1.7 g
Carbohydrate	3.3 g
Fat	1.8 g
Calcium	13.1 mg
Dietary Fiber	0.0 g

Percent of calories from:

Carbohydrate:	36%
Protein:	19%
Fat:	45%

Broccoli Apple Salad with Creamy Curry Dressing

A great winter salad, this can also serve as a filling for pitas. Or add cooked chicken for a summer main course. The curried dressing makes a great dip for veggies too!

1	bunch broccoli	1
3	apples, cored and coarsely chopped	3
2	stalks celery, sliced	2
¼ cup	sesame seeds, toasted	50 mL
1 cup	sunflower sprouts or alfalfa sprouts	250 mL

Creamy Curry Dressing

1	pkg (10.25 oz/290 g) silken soft tofu	1
2 tbsp	each fresh lemon juice and vegetable oil	25 mL
1 tbsp	granulated sugar	15 mL
1 tsp	each curry powder and salt	5 mL
¼ tsp	black pepper	1 mL

1. Creamy Curry Dressing: Using sieve, drain tofu.

2. Meanwhile, trim tough broccoli stems. Cut broccoli into florets and remaining stem into thin slices. In saucepan of rapidly boiling water, cook broccoli, uncovered, for 4 to 5 minutes or until crisp-tender. Drain and run under cold water to stop broccoli cooking.

3. In mixing bowl, combine broccoli, apples and celery.

4. In food processor, purée drained tofu, lemon juice, oil, sugar, curry powder, salt and pepper until smooth. Toss enough with salad to lightly coat. Refrigerate any remaining dressing in airtight container for up to 2 days.

5. Serve garnished with sesame seeds on bed of sunflower sprouts.

Makes 8 servings

To toast sesame seeds, arrange on baking sheet and bake in preheated 350°F (180°C) oven 10 to 12 minutes or until golden brown and fragrant.

Per serving

Salad with dressing:

Calories	130.7
Protein	4.7 g
Carbohydrate	15.9 g
Fat	6.7 g
Calcium	101.0 mg
	(a source)
Dietary Fiber	3.7 g
	(a source)

Percent of calories from:

Carbohydrate:	45%
Protein:	13%
Fat:	42%

Per serving   (1 tbsp/15 mL)

Dressing:

Calories	16.8
Protein	0.6 g
Carbohydrate	0.9 g
Fat	1.3 g
Calcium	4.5 mg
Dietary Fiber	0.0 g

Percent of calories from:

Carbohydrate:	22%
Protein:	13%
Fat:	65%

Cucumber Almond Salad

Makes 6 servings

The calcium crunch from the almonds is a delectable contrast to the freshness of the cucumber. The salad is a great partner to fish or seafood.

Almonds go soggy if combined in a salad with dressing and allowed to stand.

1	English cucumber	1
½ cup	slivered unblanched almonds	125 mL

Dressing

¼ cup	each fresh lemon juice and vegetable oil	50 mL
1 tbsp	liquid honey	15 mL
1 tsp	grated lemon rind	5 mL
½ tsp	salt	2 mL
¼ tsp	black pepper	1 mL

1. Slice cucumbers thinly, about 1/8 inch (3 mm). Set aside in bowl.

2. Preheat oven to 350°F (180°C). Toast almonds on baking sheet for 10 to 15 minutes or until golden and fragrant.

3. Dressing: In mixing bowl or food processor, combine lemon juice, oil, honey, lemon rind, salt and pepper. Pour enough over cucumbers to coat. (You may have enough for 2 salads depending on size of cucumber.)

4. To serve, sprinkle with almonds.

Per serving

Calories	151.9
Protein	2.6 g
Carbohydrate	8.8 g
Fat	12.9 g
Calcium	44.1 mg
Dietary Fiber	1.7 g

Percent of calories from:

Carbohydrate:	22%
Protein:	6%
Fat:	72%

Rossolye Salad

This colorful Russian beet and apple salad with sardines is a tasty addition to a buffet table. The calcium-containing dressing can do triple duty as a sauce for fish, a spread for sandwiches or a vegetable dip.

Makes 6 servings

1	bunch beets, washed	1
3	potatoes, peeled and quartered	3
2	apples, cored and coarsely chopped	2
1	can sardines, drained and chopped (100 g)	1
	Dill sprigs	

Creamy Dill Dressing

1	pkg (10.25 oz/290 g) silken soft tofu	1
⅓ cup	chopped fresh dill	75 mL
3 tbsp	fresh lemon juice	50 mL
2 tbsp	vegetable oil	25 mL
1 tbsp	each Dijon mustard and granulated sugar	15 mL
1 tsp	salt	5 mL
¼ tsp	black pepper	1 mL

1. Using sieve, drain tofu.

2. Meanwhile, in saucepan of rapidly boiling water, cook beets until tender, about 20 minutes. Drain and let cool enough to handle. Peel and dice into 1/2-inch (1 cm) cubes.

3. Meanwhile, in same saucepan with more water, cook potatoes until tender, about 15 minutes. Drain and dice into 1/2-inch (1 cm) cubes.

Tomato Basil Salad: Slice beefsteak or hothouse tomatoes and arrange on a platter. Drizzle with extra virgin olive oil and sprinkle with chopped fresh basil and 2 cloves minced garlic. Cover until ready to serve. Serve at room temperature.

4. In mixing bowl, combine cooled beets, potatoes and apples. Set aside.

5. In food processor with pulsing motion, combine drained tofu, dill, lemon juice, oil, mustard, sugar, salt and pepper; purée until smooth. Dressing can be refrigerated in airtight container for up to 2 days.

6. Toss salad gently with about half of the dressing or just enough to coat. Cover and refrigerate for up to 1 day. Serve garnished with sardines and dill. Pass bowl of remaining dressing separately.

Per serving

Calories	175.6
Protein	7.5 g
Carbohydrate	26.5 g
Fat	5.0 g
Calcium	109.3 mg
	(a source)
Dietary Fiber	3.3 g
	(a source)

Percent of calories from:

Carbohydrate:	59%
Protein:	17%
Fat:	25%

Salad of Fresh Spring Greens, New Potatoes and Asparagus

This beautiful salad is a true celebration of spring or summer.

12	small new potatoes, scrubbed	12
1 lb	asparagus	500 g
8 oz	fiddleheads	125 g
16 cups	assorted field greens (beet greens, watercress, Boston, leaf, romaine, arugula)	4 L
2	large hothouse tomatoes, cut in wedges	2

Herbal Vinaigrette

¼ cup	white wine vinegar	50 mL
¼ cup	each water, vegetable oil and extra virgin olive oil	50 mL
1	clove garlic, minced	1
2 tsp	chopped fresh tarragon, thyme or rosemary and Dijon mustard	10 mL
1 tsp	each salt and granulated sugar	5 mL
¼ tsp	black pepper	1 mL

1. In steamer over simmering water, steam potatoes until tender, about 15 minutes. Drain well.

2. Meanwhile, in large pot of boiling water, cook asparagus and fiddleheads until tender-crisp, 2 to 3 minutes. Drain and refresh under cold water. Cut asparagus into 2-inch (10 cm) pieces.

3. Herbal Vinaigrette: In food processor or mixing bowl using whisk, combine vinegar, water, vegetable and olive oils, garlic, tarragon, mustard, salt, sugar and pepper until smooth.

4. In large bowl, toss together greens, asparagus, fiddleheads and potatoes with enough dressing to coat. Arrange on platter or individual plates. Garnish with tomato wedges.

Makes 6 servings

This salad is wonderful as a bed for grilled salmon. Sprinkle it with herbs and serve with lemon wedges.

Per serving

Calories	361.8
Protein	9.4 g
Carbohydrate	46.5 g
Fat	16.9 g
Calcium	175.9 mg
	(a high source)
Dietary Fiber	6.3 g
	(a very high source)

Percent of calories from:

Carbohydrate:	50%
Protein:	10%
Fat:	40%

Per serving (1 tbsp/15 mL)

Vinaigrette:

Calories	57.7
Protein	0.1 g
Carbohydrate	0.9 g
Fat	6.2 g
Calcium	9.6 mg
Dietary Fiber	0.0 g

Percent of calories from:

Carbohydrate:	6%
Protein:	1%
Fat:	94%

Spring Salad with Oriental Flavors

Makes 6 servings

Tofu and sesame seeds are sources of calcium. Any leftover tofu can be frozen for future use. For variety, feel free to substitute the best veggies available—sliced bok choy, broccoli, fiddleheads or mushrooms.

1 lb	asparagus, tough ends removed	500 g
2 cups	frozen peas	500 mL
4	carrots, peeled and cut into julienne strips	4
1	small sweet red pepper, cut into strips	1
6 oz	extra firm tofu, cubed	175 g
1 tbsp	toasted sesame seeds	15 mL

Oriental Dressing

3 tbsp	vegetable oil	50 mL
3 tbsp	fresh lemon juice	50 mL
2 tbsp	liquid honey	25 mL
2 tsp	each grated fresh gingerroot and soy sauce	10 mL
1	clove garlic, minced	1
¼ tsp	salt	1 mL
Pinch	black pepper	Pinch

1. In large pot of boiling water cook asparagus, peas and carrots until tender-crisp, about 2 to 3 minutes. Drain and refresh under cold water.

2. Oriental Dressing: In small bowl, whisk together oil, lemon juice, honey, ginger, soy sauce, garlic, salt and pepper. Cover and refrigerate for up to 2 days.

3. In bowl, toss asparagus, peas, carrots, red pepper and tofu with dressing just before serving. Sprinkle with sesame seeds.

Per serving

Calories	188.4
Protein	7.8 g
Carbohydrate	20.9 g
Fat	9.1 g
Calcium	62.6 mg
	(a source)
Dietary Fiber	4.0 g
	(a high source)

Percent of calories from:

Carbohydrate:	42%
Protein:	16%
Fat:	42%

Breakfast, Brunch and Lunch

MANY NORTH AMERICANS start the day with a bowl of cereal with milk. For lactose-intolerant people, cereal must be made without lactose (read the label, see page 4) and milk should be lactose-reduced or soy milk. Here are some recipes using lactose-reduced milk, juices, stock, soy milk and tofu so you can begin your day free of symptoms.

Fruit Smoothie

This mini-meal in a glass replaces the old-fashioned eggnog and provides calcium if you use tofu made with calcium sulfate or calcium chloride. Make it with your kids' favorite fruit and serve with a color-ful straw. It's sure to be a hit.

Makes 2 drinks

1	pkg (10.25 oz/290 g) silken soft tofu	1
1 cup	fruit juice (orange, apple or cranberry)	250 mL
1	banana	1
1 cup	berries such as strawberries or blueberries (optional)	250 mL

1. In blender or food processor, purée tofu, fruit juice, banana, and berries (if using) until smooth. Pour into glasses and serve immediately.

Per serving

Calories	215.4
Protein	8.2 g
Carbohydrate	38.1 g
Fat	4.8 g
Calcium	62.6 mg
	(a source)
Dietary Fiber	2.8 g
	(a source)

Percent of calories from:

Carbohydrate:	67%
Protein:	14%
Fat:	19%

Orange French Toast

Makes 6 servings

The best part of this vibrant way to start the day is that you can prepare it the night before. The hint of liqueur raises an ordinary recipe to the sublime.

6	slices (1-inch/2.5 cm thick) French bread	6
6	eggs	6
1 cup	orange juice	250 mL
2 tbsp	grated orange rind	25 mL
2 tbsp	granulated sugar	25 mL
1 tbsp	Grand Marnier or other orange-flavored liqueur (optional)	15 mL
1 tsp	vanilla	5 mL

Orange Marmalade Sauce

½ cup	orange marmalade	125 mL
¼ cup	orange juice	50 mL
2 tbsp	honey	25 mL
1 tbsp	Grand Marnier (optional)	15 mL

If bread is already sliced thinly, use two slices stacked on top of each other.

1. In mixing bowl, beat together eggs, orange juice and rind, sugar, Grand Marnier (if using) and vanilla.

2. Arrange bread, cutting to fit, in single layer in greased 13- x 9-inch (3 L) baking dish. Pour orange mixture over top; cover and refrigerate overnight.

3. Preheat oven to 350°F (180°C). Bake, uncovered, for 25 to 30 minutes or until no longer soggy and firm to touch.

4. Orange Marmalade Sauce: Meanwhile, in saucepan, bring marmalade, orange juice and honey to boil; reduce heat and simmer, stirring, about 5 minutes or until slightly thickened. Serve with French toast.

Per serving

Calories	377.0
Protein	12.2 g
Carbohydrate	64.9 g
Fat	7.3 g
Calcium	104.8 mg (a source)
Dietary Fiber	3.0 g (a source)

Percent of calories from:

Carbohydrate:	68%
Protein:	13%
Fat:	17%

French Toastwich

Make this no-fuss dish to eat with a salad and your favorite pickle for a sure-to-please lunch or supper.

Makes 1 serving

2	slices bread	2
1 tsp	each Dijon mustard and light mayonnaise	5 mL
1 oz	shaved Black Forest ham, smoked turkey or smoked chicken	30 g
1	egg	1
1 tbsp	water	15 mL

1. Spread 1 slice of bread with mustard; spread remaining slice with mayonnaise. Sandwich ham between bread.

2. In mixing bowl, whisk together egg and water. Dip sandwich into mixture, turning to coat other side. Let stand a few minutes to absorb all liquid.

3. Heat nonstick skillet over medium-high heat; cook sandwich on both sides until golden brown and firm to touch. Cut in half and serve at once.

Per serving

Calories	374.7
Protein	20.3 g
Carbohydrate	42.0 g
Fat	13.0 g
Calcium	84.9 mg (a source)
Dietary Fiber	1.6 g

Percent of calories from:

Carbohydrate:	46%
Protein:	22%
Fat:	32%

Apple French Toastwich

Makes 1 serving

A variation on an old theme, this version is tasty with a dab of honey-mustard or fruit chutney. It doubles for breakfast or a light supper.

2	slices raisin bread	2
1 tsp	each Dijon mustard and mayonnaise	5 mL
1 oz	shaved Black Forest ham, smoked turkey or smoked chicken	30 g
Quarter	apple, peeled, sliced and cored	Quarter
1	egg	1
1 tbsp	water	15 mL

1. Spread 1 slice of bread with mustard; spread remaining slice with mayonnaise. Sandwich ham and apple between bread.

2. In mixing bowl, whisk together egg and water. Dip sandwich into mixture, turning to coat each side. Let stand a few minutes to absorb all liquid.

3. Heat nonstick skillet over medium-high heat; cook sandwich on both sides until golden brown and firm to touch. Cut in half and serve at once.

To make a strata: A strata is basically baked French toast. Try making your favorite sandwich, such as salmon salad, then pour beaten egg and water, lactose-reduced milk or soy milk over sandwich. Cover and refrigerate. The next day cook in a heated skillet or bake in a 350°F (180°C) oven for 40 to 45 minutes or until puffed and firm to touch.

Per serving

Calories	316.3
Protein	17.6 g
Carbohydrate	32.7 g
Fat	12.6 g
Calcium	81.7 mg
	(a source)
Dietary Fiber	1.5 g

Percent of calories from:

Carbohydrate:	42%
Protein:	22%
Fat:	36%

Make-Ahead Scramble

This is a variation of a popular egg casserole that I like to make for brunch because I can assemble it the night before. In the original, the cheese sauce helps keep the eggs moist for advance preparation. In this recipe, a tofu cream sauce and flavorful olive oil do the duty of cheese sauce with no lactose, less fat and lots of taste!

1 tbsp	extra virgin olive oil	15 mL
4 oz	mushrooms, sliced	125 g
3	green onions, chopped	3
8	eggs, beaten	8

Tofu Cream Sauce

1	pkg (10.25 oz/290 g) silken soft tofu	1
2 tbsp	light mayonnaise	25 mL
1 tbsp	fresh lemon juice	15 mL
1 tbsp	freshly grated Parmesan cheese (optional, if tolerated)	15 mL
1/4 tsp	salt	1 mL
Pinch	each black pepper and nutmeg	Pinch

Herbed Crumb Topping

1 cup	dry bread crumbs	250 mL
¼ cup	chopped fresh parsley	50 mL
1 tbsp	extra virgin olive oil	15 mL
1 tbsp	freshly grated Parmesan cheese (optional, if tolerated)	15 mL
¼ tsp	dried thyme	1 mL

Makes 4 servings

Per serving

Calories	408.5
Protein	22.6 g
Carbohydrate	27.4 g
Fat	24.0 g
Calcium	213.9 mg
	(a high source)
Dietary Fiber	3.2 g
	(a source)

Percent of calories from:

Carbohydrate:	26%
Protein:	22%
Fat:	52%

Add 4 oz (125 g) chopped smoked ham or salmon just before spooning into pie plate.

Store fresh mushrooms in refrigerator for up to 1 week in paper bag rather than in plastic, where they are too moist and become slimy.

1. Tofu Cream Sauce: Using sieve, drain tofu.

2. In large skillet, heat oil over medium heat; cook mushrooms and green onions for 5 minutes or until softened.

3. Add eggs; cook, stirring, for 5 to 7 minutes or until eggs are just set. Remove from heat.

4. In mixing bowl or food processor, beat together drained tofu, mayonnaise, lemon juice, cheese (if using), salt, pepper and nutmeg until smooth. Stir into eggs until well combined. Spoon into greased 10-inch (1.5 L) pie plate.

5. Herbed Crumb Topping: In mixing bowl, combine bread crumbs, parsley, oil, cheese (if using) and thyme; sprinkle over eggs. Cover and refrigerate up to 12 hours.

6. Preheat oven to 350°F (180°C). Bake for 25 to 30 minutes or until heated through. Serve immediately.

Dilled Salmon Soufflé

If you want a simple recipe with a touch of glamor, try this soufflé. You can use sockeye or the less expensive pink salmon if you prefer. Remember to crush and include the bones for added calcium. Serve with crusty bread and a green salad for a quick but tasty treat.

1	can (7.5 oz/213 g) salmon	1
6	eggs, separated	6
1 cup	fresh bread crumbs	250 mL
2 tbsp	fresh lemon juice	25 mL
2 tbsp	chopped fresh dill	25 mL
1 tsp	Worcestershire sauce	5 mL
½ tsp	salt	2 mL
½ tsp	dry mustard	2 mL
Pinch	cayenne pepper	Pinch

1. Preheat oven to 400°F (200°C).

2. Drain salmon; discard skin, reserving bones. In mixing bowl, beat together salmon with bones, 5 egg yolks, bread crumbs, lemon juice, dill, Worcestershire sauce, salt, mustard and cayenne pepper until well combined. Set aside.

3. In separate bowl and using clean beaters, beat 6 egg whites until in stiff peaks. Fold about one-third into salmon mixture to lighten. Gently fold in remaining egg white.

4. Spoon into ungreased 6-cup (1.5 L) soufflé dish or straight-sided baking dish. Bake for 25 to 30 minutes or until set but center still a little moist. Serve immediately.

Makes 4 servings

To judge whether egg whites are stiff enough once beaten, turn bowl almost upside down. If egg white stays intact and inside, they are stiff.

Leftover egg yolks can be covered and refrigerated for a day. Mixed with a spoonful of water, they can be painted on breads, cookies and pastry to give a golden sheen. They can be saved to make scrambled eggs or used to make a custard. If all else fails, feed them to your pet cat or dog. They are sure to appreciate the treat.

Per serving

Calories	303.1
Protein	22.0 g
Carbohydrate	20.5 g
Fat	14.3 g
Calcium	215.4 mg
	(a high source)
Dietary Fiber	0.9 g

Percent of calories from:

Carbohydrate:	27%
Protein:	29%
Fat:	43%

Potato Tortilla

Makes 4 servings

This simple dish takes you on a quick trip to Spain. Serve the tortilla with crusty bread, olives, sliced tomato salad and Rioja wine.

3	large potatoes, peeled and quartered	3
2 tbsp	extra virgin olive oil	25 mL
1	onion, chopped	1
1	clove garlic, minced	1
3	eggs	3
1 cup	fresh bread crumbs	250 mL
½ cup	chicken stock	125 mL
¼ cup	chopped fresh parsley	50 mL
½ tsp	salt	2 mL
¼ tsp	each black pepper and nutmeg	1 mL

Seasoned Bread Crumbs

1 cup	fresh bread crumbs	250 mL
¼ cup	chopped fresh parsley	50 mL
1 tbsp	extra virgin olive oil	15 mL
1 tbsp	freshly grated Parmesan cheese (optional, if tolerated)	15 mL
¼ tsp	each black pepper and dried thyme	1 mL

1. Preheat oven to 350°F (180°C). In steamer over simmering water, cook potatoes 15 to 20 minutes or until just tender. Cool and cube.

2. In skillet, heat oil over medium-high heat; cook onion and garlic, covered, 5 minutes until soft.

3. In mixing bowl, whisk together eggs, bread crumbs, chicken stock, parsley, salt, pepper and nutmeg. Stir in cubed potatoes and onion mixture. Spoon into greased 9-inch (1 L) pie plate.

4. Seasoned Bread Crumbs: In small bowl, toss together bread crumbs, parsley, oil, cheese (if using), pepper and thyme; sprinkle over potato mixture.

5. Bake 40 to 45 minutes until set. Let stand 15 minutes before cutting into wedges. Can be covered and refrigerated overnight. Serve hot or room temperature.

Per serving

Calories	483.4
Protein	15.4 g
Carbohydrate	69.5 g
Fat	16.3 g
Calcium	132.0 mg
	(a source)
Dietary Fiber	5.4 g
	(a high source)

Percent of calories from:

Carbohydrate:	57%
Protein:	13%
Fat:	30%

Orange Pancakes

The secret to these tender pancakes is cake-and-pastry flour. They may be served with the usual maple syrup or spread with marmalade. You won't miss butter. To make a mini sandwich, use a tablespoon of batter to make each pancake and spread with Tofu Cream Cheese (page 168) and marmalade. It's the perfect size for a child's breakfast or snack.

2 cups	cake-and-pastry flour	500 mL
¼ cup	granulated sugar	50 mL
2 tsp	baking powder	10 mL
½ tsp	baking soda	2 mL
½ tsp	salt	2 mL
1 cup	orange juice	250 mL
3 tbsp	vegetable oil	50 mL
1	egg	1

1. In mixing bowl, sift together flour, sugar, baking powder, baking soda and salt.

2. In measuring cup whisk together orange juice, oil and egg. Pour into dry ingredients, stirring with fork just until dry ingredients are moistened.

3. Heat nonstick skillet over medium-high heat. For each pancake, spoon 1/4 cup (50 mL) batter into pan. Cook until bubbles appear and break. Flip and cook until second side is golden brown. Serve at once.

Makes about twelve 4-inch/10 cm pancakes

To store pancakes, stack separated with waxed paper, double-wrap stack in foil and refrigerate up to 2 days or freeze up to 3 months. Defrost in the refrigerator overnight and reheat in the microwave or toaster.

Orange juice replaces the usual milk in this recipe. For a variation, try apple juice instead and use half whole wheat flour with a pinch of cinnamon instead of all cake-and-pastry flour. Serve with apple butter (page 165).

Per serving (1 pancake)

Calories	125.4
Protein	2.1 g
Carbohydrate	19.9 g
Fat	4.0 g
Calcium	8.2 mg
Dietary Fiber	0.5 g

Percent of calories from:

Carbohydrate:	64%
Protein:	7%
Fat:	29%

Basic Crêpes

Makes 10 to 16 crêpes or about 30 mini-crêpes

For a quick dessert idea, squeeze fresh lemon juice over large crêpe, sprinkle with granulated sugar and fold into quarters. Serve with sliced fresh strawberries, blueberries or raspberries.

For a savory hors d'oeuvre, spoon a dab of your favorite sandwich filling (salmon, tuna) onto mini-crêpe and garnish with chopped green onions or dill sprig.

For a delicious main course, fill the large crêpes with creamy mushroom and chicken filling (see Chicken Pot Pie recipe page 104) and roll up.

Per serving (1 of 10 crêpes)

Calories	92.4
Protein	3.8 g
Carbohydrate	11.8 g
Fat	3.2 g
Calcium	51.9 mg
Dietary Fiber	0.4 g

Percent of calories from:

Carbohydrate:	52%
Protein:	16%
Fat:	32%

Somehow crêpes always seem special. They can be filled with a sweet or savory filling—a great way of using up leftovers. It's worth making a batch and keeping some in the freezer for emergencies. Just wrap in plastic wrap, separating each crêpe with a piece of waxed paper and double-wrapping in foil to protect them from freezer burn. They will keep frozen for up to three months.

1 cup	all-purpose flour	250 mL
1 tsp	granulated sugar	5 mL
½ tsp	salt	2 mL
1½ cups	lactose-reduced milk or soy milk	375 mL
2	eggs	2
1 tbsp	vegetable oil	15 mL

1. In mixing bowl, stir together flour, sugar and salt.

2. In measuring cup, whisk together milk, eggs and oil; pour into dry ingredients and whisk until smooth. Cover and refrigerate at least 1 hour or overnight.

3. Spray nonstick skillet with nonstick baking spray; heat over medium-high heat.

4. For each crêpe, spoon 2 tbsp (25 mL) batter into pan for 5-inch (10 cm) appetizer-size crêpe, 1/4 cup (50 mL) for dessert or dinner-size crêpe, tilting pan to coat bottom. Cook until pale brown around edges and starting to pull away from pan. Flip and cook until second side is browned.

5. Stack crêpes on plate, separating with pieces of waxed paper. Crêpes can be covered and refrigerated for up to 1 day.

Yeast Blini

These savory pancakes may be served at breakfast, lunch or dinner. Make mini ones and serve with Tofu Cream Cheese (page 168) and caviar or smoked salmon as an appetizer. Or make them full-size and serve with Quick Strawberry Sauce or the blueberry variation (page 208).

Makes about sixteen (4-inch/10cm) blini or about 30 mini ones

½ cup	lukewarm water	125 mL
1 tbsp	active dry yeast (1 pkg)	15 mL
2 tsp	granulated sugar	10 mL
1 cup	all-purpose flour	250 mL
¾ cup	lukewarm beer, lactose-reduced milk or soy milk	175 mL
½ cup	whole wheat flour	125 mL
2	eggs, beaten	2
2 tbsp	vegetable oil	25 mL
½ tsp	salt	2 mL

1. Rinse large bowl with hot water; dry well. Pour in lukewarm water; sprinkle yeast and sugar over water. Let stand in warm place 10 minutes or until yeast is foamy.

2. Gradually whisk in all-purpose flour, beer, whole wheat flour, eggs, oil and salt until smooth.

3. Cover bowl with plastic wrap; set bowl in pan of warm water until batter has doubled in size, about 1 hour. Stir down batter.

4. Heat nonstick skillet over medium-high heat. For each blini, spoon 1 tbsp (15 mL) batter for mini size, 1/4 cup (50 mL) batter for larger size into skillet; cook about 1 minute or until bubbles break on top and underside is golden brown. Flip and cook until second side is golden brown.

Per serving (1/16th)

Calories	71.4
Protein	2.3 g
Carbohydrate	9.9 g
Fat	2.2 g
Calcium	6.8 mg
Dietary Fiber	0.9 g

Percent of calories from:

Carbohydrate:	55%
Protein:	13%
Fat:	28%

Main Courses

Pasta and Pizza

PASTA AND PIZZA frequently include cheese toppings or cream sauces with accompanying bowls of cheese. By using a minimum of Parmesan cheese, an aged hard cheese, seasoned bread crumbs for topping and rich sauces made from lactose-reduced milk, pasta and pizza can still appear on the menu. Those with lactose intolerance will have to find their individual tolerance level for cheese. Hard aged cheeses, low in lactose, like Parmesan, Cheddar and Swiss may be digested comfortably, especially if consumed in small quantities.

Garden Lasagne

Feel free to substitute any green or white vegetables you have in abundance. A combination of leek, broccoli, spinach, beans, zucchini, green pepper, cauliflower or mushrooms are all possibilities that work well to make about 14 cups (3.5 L) of chopped prepared vegetables before cooking. The packaged fresh pasta noodles are a great time-saver in this recipe, because they require no pre-cooking.

Makes 8 servings

1	bunch broccoli	1
1	bag (10 oz/284 g) fresh spinach	1
1	bunch leeks (white part only) (2 or 3)	1
1	head cauliflower	1
8 oz	mushrooms, sliced	250 g
3	cloves garlic, minced	3
2 tbsp	extra virgin olive oil	25 mL
1 tsp	each dried basil and tarragon	5 mL
¼ tsp	black pepper	1 mL
1	pkg (12 oz/350 g) fresh lasagne pasta	1

Béchamel Tofu Sauce

2	pkg (10.25 oz/290 g) silken soft tofu	2
¼ cup	chopped fresh parsley	50 mL
2 tbsp	extra virgin olive oil	25 mL
1 tbsp	Dijon mustard	15 mL
1 tbsp	freshly grated Parmesan cheese (optional, if tolerated)	15 mL
½ tsp	salt	2 mL
¼ tsp	each black pepper and nutmeg	1 mL
2	eggs	2

Seasoned Bread Crumbs

1 cup	fresh bread crumbs (preferably from Italian-style bread)	250 mL
¼ cup	chopped fresh parsley	50 mL
1 tbsp	freshly grated Parmesan cheese (optional, if tolerated)	15 mL
1 tbsp	extra-virgin olive oil	15 mL
¼ tsp	each dried thyme, black pepper and salt	1 mL

1. Trim broccoli stems and slice stalks; cut broccoli into florets. Trim spinach stems. Clean leeks and slice thinly. Cut cauliflower into florets. Rinse all vegetables under water, shaking off excess.

2. Using 24-cup (6 L) Dutch oven, and with about 1 cup (250 mL) water, cover and cook broccoli, spinach, leeks, cauliflower, mushrooms, garlic, olive oil, basil, tarragon and pepper, in two batches, until florets are crisp-tender and spinach is wilted, about 5 minutes, adding more water as necessary to prevent burning. Set aside.

3. Béchamel Tofu Sauce: Meanwhile, using sieve, drain tofu.

4. In food processor using pulsing motion, purée drained tofu, parsley, oil, mustard, cheese (if using), salt, pepper, nutmeg and eggs until smooth.

5. Seasoned Bread Crumbs: In mixing bowl, stir together bread crumbs, parsley, cheese (if using), olive oil, thyme, pepper and salt.

6. Preheat oven to 350°F (180°C). Grease 13- x 9-inch (3 L) baking dish.

7. To assemble lasagne, sprinkle about 1 cup (250 mL) vegetable mixture on bottom of casserole. Cover with layer of 2 lasagne sheets. Spread half of the remaining vegetables over top. Cover with 2 more pastas sheets. Spread remaining vegetables over pasta. Top with 2 more pasta sheets. Spread Béchamel Tofu Sauce over top. Sprinkle evenly with Seasoned Bread Crumbs.

8. Bake, uncovered, for 25 to 30 minutes or until heated through. Let stand for 15 minutes before cutting into squares.

Look for fresh lasagne noodles (sheets) in the refrigerated deli section of the grocery store.

Per serving

Lasagne:

Calories	466.9
Protein	19.6 g
Carbohydrate	66.5 g
Fat	14.9 g
Calcium	194.8 mg
	(a high source)
Dietary Fiber	7.4 g
	(a very high source)

Percent of calories from:

Carbohydrate:	56%
Protein:	16%
Fat:	28%

Linguine with Creamy Mushroom and Ham Sauce

Makes 4 servings

This is a favorite in our house because it's quick and simple to do and has a wonderful richness, like cream, but with very little fat. It's special enough to serve for company.

Allow 12 to 16 oz (375 to 500 g) pasta for four servings.

2 tbsp	extra virgin olive oil	25 mL
1	onion, chopped	1
1	clove garlic, minced	1
12 oz	mushrooms, sliced	375 g
¼ cup	dry sherry or white wine	50 mL
1 tsp	dried thyme	5 mL
¼ tsp	nutmeg	1 mL
2 tbsp	all-purpose flour	25 mL
2 cups	lactose-reduced milk or soy milk	500 mL
1 cup	chopped Black Forest ham or smoked turkey	250 mL
½ tsp	salt	2 mL
¼ tsp	black pepper	1 mL
¼ cup	chopped fresh parsley	50 mL
1 lb	linguine	500 g

1. In large skillet, heat oil over medium heat; cook onion and garlic for 5 to 8 minutes or until softened.

2. Add mushrooms, sherry, thyme and nutmeg; cook, uncovered, about 5 minutes or until mushrooms release juices.

3. Sprinkle with flour, stirring to combine. Gradually whisk in milk; cook, stirring, until smooth and thickened. Stir in ham, salt, pepper and parsley.

4. Meanwhile, cook pasta. Drain and serve immediately tossed with sauce.

Per serving

Calories	671.3
Protein	29.0 g
Carbohydrate	102.2 g
Fat	14.5 g
Calcium	204.1 mg
	(a high source)
Dietary Fiber	5.9 g
	(a high source)

Percent of calories from:

Carbohydrate:	61%
Protein:	17%
Fat:	19%

Tuna Vegetable Sauce

Remember that much-loved tuna casserole? Here's a revamped version using soy milk to make a speedy sauce for noodles or rice the whole family can enjoy.

1 tbsp	vegetable oil	15 mL
2 cups	sliced mushrooms (8 oz/250 g)	500 mL
1	stalk celery, chopped (½ cup/125 mL)	1
1	small onion, chopped (½ cup/125 mL)	1
⅓	chopped sweet red or green pepper,	75 mL
1	clove garlic, minced	1
1 tbsp	all-purpose flour	15 mL
1½ cups	soy milk or lactose-reduced milk	375 mL
1	can (6.5 oz/184 g) tuna packed in water, drained	1
1 tbsp	ketchup	15 mL
1 tsp	Worcestershire sauce	5 mL
½ tsp	salt	2 mL
¼ cup	chopped fresh parsley	50 mL

1. In large saucepan, heat oil over medium heat; cook mushrooms, celery, onion, red pepper and garlic, covered, 8 to 10 minutes or until onions are softened.

2. Sprinkle with flour, stirring to combine. Gradually stir in soy milk; cook, stirring, over medium heat until thickened.

3. Stir in tuna, ketchup, Worcestershire sauce and salt until well combined. Spoon over rice or pasta; sprinkle with parsley.

Makes about 3 cups (750 mL)

Cook rice or pasta according to package directions. Allow 2 cups uncooked parboiled rice for 4 servings and 12 oz to 1 lb (375 to 500 g) pasta for 4 servings.

Per serving
(3/4 cup/175 mL)

Calories	160.3
Protein	17.4 g
Carbohydrate	11.0 g
Fat	5.7 g
Calcium	33.0 mg
Dietary Fiber	3.0 g
	(a source)

Percent of calories from:

Carbohydrate:	27%
Protein:	42%
Fat:	31%

Fettuccini Alfredo

Makes 4 servings

To me, this is the ultimate luxury food—fast, rich and soothing. This lactose-free version is lower in fat than the original made with whipping cream, a bonus to be enjoyed without guilt!

2 tbsp	extra virgin olive oil	25 mL
1	shallot, chopped	1
1	clove garlic, minced	1
2 tbsp	all-purpose flour	25 mL
2½ cups	2% lactose-reduced milk	625 mL
1	bay leaf	1
½ tsp	salt	2 mL
¼ tsp	each black pepper and grated nutmeg	1 mL
12 oz	fettuccini	375 g
	Freshly grated Parmesan cheese (optional, if tolerated)	

1. In large saucepan, heat oil over medium heat; cook shallot and garlic about 5 minutes until softened.

2. Sprinkle with flour; cook, stirring, until pale brown, about 3 minutes. Remove from heat.

3. Meanwhile, in separate saucepan, heat milk and bay leaf until bubbles appear around edge of pan. Gradually whisk about half into flour until smooth and thickened.

4. Return flour mixture to heat. Gradually whisk in remaining milk; cook, stirring, until thickened. Whisk in salt, pepper and nutmeg. Discard bay leaf.

5. Cook fettuccini according to package directions, 6 to 8 minutes or until al dente. Drain and toss with sauce. Serve sprinkled with cheese (if using).

Per serving

Calories	468.4
Protein	16.5 g
Carbohydrate	74.7 g
Fat	11.1 g
Calcium	207.7 mg
	(a high source)
Dietary Fiber	2.2 g

Percent of calories from:

Carbohydrate:	64%
Protein:	14%
Fat:	22%

Macaroni and Cheese

Warm and comforting, macaroni and cheese is as popular with toddlers as with adults. Lactose-reduced milk adds natural sweetness and creaminess to the dish. Aged firm cheeses such as Cheddar, Swiss, Gouda and Parmesan are often better digested by lactose-intolerant people because they are low in lactose. Use only if tolerated.

Makes 4 servings, about 6 cups (1.5 L)

2 cups	elbow macaroni	500 mL
1 tsp	salt	5 mL

Sauce

4 cups	lactose-reduced milk	1 L
¼ cup	vegetable oil	50 mL
¼ cup	all-purpose flour	50 mL
1	bay leaf	1
2 tsp	each Dijon mustard and Worcestershire sauce	10 mL
	Salt and pepper	
2 cups	shredded old Cheddar cheese (if tolerated)	500 mL

Bread Crumbs

¼ cup	dry bread crumbs	50 mL
1 tbsp	each extra virgin olive oil, freshly grated Parmesan cheese (if tolerated) and chopped fresh parsley	15 mL

1. Preheat oven to 350°F (180°C). Grease 6-cup (1.5 L) baking dish.

2. In large pot of boiling water, cook macaroni and salt for 8 minutes or until al dente (tender but firm). Drain.

Using hot milk to make a béchamel sauce speeds up its thickening and makes it easier to keep smooth.

Soy milk, instead of lactose-reduced milk, can be used to make a béchamel sauce. However, the flavor is flat and the beige color requires more parsley.

If Cheddar cheese is not tolerated in the quantity suggested in the recipe substitute 1/4 cup to 1/2 cup (50 mL to 125 mL) freshly grated Parmesan cheese depending on your tolerance level.

3. Sauce: Meanwhile, in saucepan, heat milk over medium heat with bay leaf until bubbles appear around edge of pan, about 4 minutes.

4. Meanwhile, heat oil over medium heat in another saucepan. Stir in flour, cooking until it starts to turn pale brown and pull away from side of pan. Gradually whisk in heated milk, cooking until thickened and smooth, about 5 minutes. Whisk in mustard and Worcestershire sauce. Season with salt and pepper to taste. Stir in cheese. Discard bay leaf.

5. Stir in macaroni until combined. Spoon into prepared baking dish.

6. Bread Crumbs: In small bowl, stir together bread crumbs, oil, cheese (if using) and parsley; sprinkle evenly over macaroni.

7. Bake for 30 to 35 minutes or until bubbly and browned on top.

Per serving

Calories	769.0
Protein	36.0 g
Carbohydrate	70.0 g
Fat	36.7 g
Calcium	344.0 mg
	(a very high source)
Dietary Fiber	1.8 g

Percent of calories from:

Carbohydrate:	37%
Protein:	19%
Fat:	44%

Creamy Leek and Tomato Pasta

Leeks are abundant during the winter months and jazz up weekday meals. Remember, they need careful washing because they are grown in sand, making their inner layers gritty.

Makes 4 servings

2 tbsp	extra virgin olive oil	25 mL
3	leeks (white parts only), sliced thinly	3
2	tomatoes	2
1 tsp	dried oregano	5 mL
¼ tsp	dried sage	1 mL
2 tbsp	all-purpose flour	25 mL
1 cup	chicken stock	250 mL
1 cup	lactose-reduced milk	250 mL
	Salt and pepper	
1 lb	rigatoni, fusilli or radiatore	500 g
	Freshly grated Parmesan cheese (optional, if tolerated)	

The easiest way to clean leeks is to chop off the tough green stem, leaving the white tender root. Slit this lengthwise almost to the root end then wash under cold running water.

1. In large saucepan, heat oil over medium heat; cook leeks, covered, until softened.

2. Meanwhile, in mixing bowl, pour boiling water over tomatoes. Let stand about 3 minutes. Drain and run under cold water; slip off skins. Cut each tomato into 8 wedges.

3. Sprinkle oregano and sage over leeks; stir in. Sprinkle with flour; cook, stirring, until flour is pale brown.

4. Gradually whisk in chicken stock; cook, stirring until thickened. Stir in milk, tomatoes, and salt and pepper to taste; cook until heated through.

5. Cook pasta according to package directions; drain and toss with sauce. Serve sprinkled with cheese (if using).

Per serving

Calories	742.1
Protein	25.1 g
Carbohydrate	134.3 g
Fat	11.4 g
Calcium	144.2 mg
	(a source)
Dietary Fiber	8.7 g
	(a very high source)

Percent of calories from:

Carbohydrate:	73%
Protein:	14%
Fat:	14%

Pesto Pasta

Makes 4 servings

For an instant gourmet dinner, serve this emergency pasta dish with a green salad, hot crusty bread and chilled crisp white wine. You cannot go wrong!

12 oz	fusilli pasta	375 g
	Parsley Pesto (page 33)	
1 cup	freshly grated Parmesan cheese (optional, if tolerated)	250 mL

1. In large saucepan of boiling salted water, cook pasta 8 to 10 minutes or until al dente.

2. Drain and toss with pesto. Serve with cheese (if using).

Per serving

Calories	564.8
Protein	23.5 g
Carbohydrate	67.0 g
Fat	22.4 g
Calcium	444.8 mg
	(a very high source)
Dietary Fiber	4.5 g
	(a high source)

Percent of calories from:

Carbohydrate:	48%
Protein:	17%
Fat:	36%

Far East Noodles

Speedy enough for a weeknight meal, this exotic "dinner in a dish" can double as buffet fare. Extra firm tofu combined with sesame seeds, broccoli and bok choy all contribute to the calcium content in this recipe. If your tastebuds like more kick, then spice up the dish with a dash or two of Chinese chili sauce.

Makes 4 servings

8 oz	asparagus	250 g
2 cups	broccoli florets	500 mL
2 tbsp	vegetable oil	25 mL
12 oz	chicken breast or pork tenderloin, cut into strips	375 g
12 oz	extra firm tofu, cut into 1/2-inch (1 cm) cubes	375 g
2 cups	each sliced bok choy and mushrooms	500 mL
Half	sweet red pepper, sliced	Half
6	green onions, chopped	6
2 tbsp	grated fresh gingerroot	25 mL
2	cloves garlic, crushed	2
1	pkg (12 oz/375 g) Cantonese Chinese precooked noodles	1
2 tbsp	each toasted sesame seeds and chopped fresh coriander	25 mL

Sauce

½ cup	chicken stock	125 mL
¼ cup	dry sherry or rice wine vinegar	50 mL
3 tbsp	soy sauce	50 mL
2 tsp	cornstarch	10 mL
1 tsp	sesame oil	5 mL

Look for the precooked Cantonese noodles in the refrigerator counter of the meat or deli section of the grocery store.

1. Wash asparagus and break off tough ends; cut stalks into 2-inch (5 cm) diagonal pieces.

2. In Dutch oven or wok, heat about 1 inch (2.5 cm) water to boiling. Add asparagus and broccoli; cook, uncovered, about 2 minutes. Drain and set aside.

3. In same pan, heat oil over medium-high heat; cook chicken or pork about 2 minutes or until lightly brown and no longer pink. Sprinkle with tofu cubes, bok choy, mushrooms, red pepper, onions, ginger, garlic and asparagus mixture; cover and keep warm while preparing sauce.

4. Sauce: In measuring cup, whisk together chicken stock, sherry, soy sauce, cornstarch and sesame oil; pour over mixture in pan. Bring to boil and simmer, uncovered, 2 to 3 minutes or until sauce has thickened slightly and vegetables are tender-crisp. Stir mixture to coat with sauce.

5. Meanwhile, bring kettle to boil. Pull noodles apart and place in large mixing bowl. Pour boiling water over noodles: let stand 4 to 5 minutes. Drain.

6. Arrange noodles on platter or individual serving dishes. Spoon meat mixture over noodles. Sprinkle with sesame seeds and coriander.

Per serving

Calories	625.3
Protein	28.3 g
Carbohydrate	94.5 g
Fat	14.5 g
Calcium	260.5 mg
	(a high source)
Dietary Fiber	5.6 g
	(a high source)

Percent of calories from:
Carbohydrate:	59%
Protein:	18%
Fat:	21%

Florentine Lasagne

This version is so bursting with flavor that no one will ever miss the usual quantities of cheese in the traditional dish. Fresh pasta sheets speed up preparation. In fact, as a convenience, the sauce can be made ahead and frozen to use either as a pasta sauce or for the lasagne.

Makes 8 servings

1 lb	lean ground beef	500 g
2	cloves garlic, chopped	2
1	onion, chopped	1
8 oz	mushrooms, sliced (about 2½ cups/625 mL)	250 g
Half	sweet green pepper, chopped	Half
2 tsp	dried basil	10 mL
1	can (28 oz/796 mL) tomatoes	1
1	can (5.5 oz/156 mL) tomato paste	1
1 tsp	each liquid honey and salt	5 mL
¼ tsp	black pepper	1 mL
1	pkg (12 oz/350 g) fresh lasagne pasta	1

Béchamel Sauce

2 tbsp	vegetable oil	25 mL
¼ cup	all-purpose flour	50 mL
1½ cups	lactose-reduced milk	375 mL
1	bay leaf	1
¼ tsp	salt	1 mL
Pinch	each black pepper and grated nutmeg	Pinch
1 tbsp	freshly grated Parmesan cheese (optional, if tolerated)	15 mL

If you prefer, you can make the Béchamel Tofu Sauce in the Garden Lasagne (page 82) to replace this béchamel sauce.

Bread Crumb Topping

½ cup	fine dry bread crumbs	125 mL
2 tbsp	extra virgin olive oil	25 mL
2 tbsp	chopped fresh parsley	25 mL
1 tbsp	freshly grated Parmesan cheese (optional, if tolerated)	15 mL

1. In Dutch oven or large saucepan, over medium-high heat, brown beef with garlic and onion until onion is softened, about 5 minutes.

2. Stir in mushrooms, green pepper and basil; cook over medium-high about 5 minutes or until mushrooms release liquid. Stir in tomatoes and tomato paste, breaking up tomatoes; cook 10 minutes longer. Season with honey, salt and pepper.

3. Béchamel Sauce: In large heavy saucepan, stir oil with flour; cook, stirring, until pale brown. Gradually stir in milk and bay leaf; cook, stirring, over medium heat until thickened and smooth, 8 to 10 minutes. Stir in salt, pepper, nutmeg and cheese (if using). Discard bay leaf.

4. Bread Crumb Topping: In small bowl, stir together bread crumbs, oil, parsley, and cheese (if using).

5. Preheat oven to 350°F (180°C). Grease 13- x 9-inch (3 L) baking dish or spray with nonstick baking spray.

6. To assemble lasagne, spread about 2 cups (500 mL) meat sauce on bottom of baking dish. Arrange 2 sheets of pasta over sauce. Spread half of the remaining sauce over pasta. Top with 2 more sheets. Spread remaining sauce over pasta. Top with 2 more sheets of pasta. Spread béchamel sauce over top. Sprinkle with bread crumb topping.

7. Bake for 30 to 35 minutes or until heated through. Let stand for 15 minutes before cutting into squares. Lasagne may be covered and refrigerated for up to 12 hours; reheat to serve.

Per serving

Florentine Lasagne:

Calories	390.9
Protein	19.2 g
Carbohydrate	40.1 g
Fat	18.1 g
Calcium	143.3 mg
	(a source)
Dietary Fiber	4.6 g
	(a high source)

Percent of calories from:

Carbohydrate:	40%
Protein:	19%
Fat:	41%

Pesto Pizza

A supply of homemade parsley pesto is my favorite emergency staple. I try to have a jar in the freezer at all times. It's great for appetizers (Sun-Dried Tomato and Parsley Pesto dip (page 33)), it makes a wonderful pasta topping and it never fails to please pizza lovers. With a bare sprinkling of cheese, it's lip-smacking good!

Makes one 12-inch
(30 cm) pizza

	Parsley Pesto (page 33)	
1	12-inch (30 cm) prebaked pizza shell	1
2	large tomatoes, sliced	2
1 cup	freshly grated Parmesan cheese (optional, if tolerated)	250 mL

Kitchen scissors work well to cut pizza into neat wedges.

1. Preheat oven to 425°F (220°C).

2. Spread pesto on pizza shell. Arrange sliced tomatoes across surface.

3. Bake on baking sheet for 20 to 25 minutes or until heated through. Sprinkle evenly with cheese (if using). Cut into wedges to serve.

Per serving (1/6th)

Calories	401.6
Protein	15.3 g
Carbohydrate	39.2 g
Fat	19.1 g
Calcium	341.1 mg
	(a very high source)
Dietary Fiber	1.7 g

Percent of calories from:

Carbohydrate:	43%
Protein:	17%
Fat:	40%

Bruschetta Pizza

Makes one 12-inch
(30 cm) pizza

For added protein and calcium, sprinkle pizza with the marinated crumbled tofu. Serve it piping hot or at room temperature for packed lunches.

1	pkg (12 oz/350 g) pizza dough	1
2 tsp	extra virgin olive oil	10 mL
½ tsp	dried rosemary	2 mL

Topping

2	large tomatoes, chopped (2 cups/500 mL)	2
½ cup	chopped red onion	125 mL
¼ cup	chopped fresh parsley	50 mL
2	cloves garlic, minced	2
2 tbsp	extra virgin olive oil	25 mL
2 tsp	dried basil	10 mL
½ tsp	salt	2 mL

Marinated Tofu (optional)

6 oz	extra firm tofu, crumbled	175 g
1 tbsp	extra virgin olive oil	15 mL
2 tsp	balsamic vinegar	10 mL
1 tsp	dried rosemary	5 mL
	Grated Parmesan cheese (optional)	

1. Preheat oven to 450°F (230°C). Grease 12-inch (30 cm) pizza pan or spray with nonstick baking spray.

2. Marinated Tofu: In mixing bowl, combine tofu, oil, vinegar and rosemary. Let stand about 10 minutes.

3. Meanwhile, roll dough out on floured surface to fit pizza pan. Brush with oil; sprinkle with rosemary. Bake about 5 minutes or until pale brown.

4. Topping: Meanwhile, combine tomatoes, onion, parsley, garlic, oil, basil and salt.

5. Sprinkle partially baked shell evenly with topping and marinated tofu (if using). Bake about 20 minutes or until golden brown on bottom. Remove from oven and sprinkle with Parmesan cheese if tolerated.

If you are running short on time, use a purchased 12-inch (30 cm) pizza shell; brush with olive oil and sprinkle with rosemary. Sprinkle with toppings and bake at 425°F (220°C) 20 to 25 minutes or until heated through. Pizza dough is available in the deli refrigerator counters of the supermarket.

Per serving   (1/6th)

Calories	316.9
Protein	9.9 g
Carbohydrate	42.5 g
Fat	11.5 g
Calcium	34.1 mg
Dietary Fiber	1.6 g

Percent of calories from:
Carbohydrate:	54%
Protein:	13%
Fat:	33%

Four Onion Pizza with Rosemary

Makes one 12-inch
(30 cm) pizza

Onions and their relatives, shallots, garlic and leeks, become as sweet as candy when slowly sautéed. Sprinkle with a little fresh or dried herbs and you have a mouth-watering pizza.

By sprinkling cheese on pizza as it comes out of the oven, it melts nicely without being tough and chewy as it would have been if baked in the oven.

2 tbsp	extra virgin olive oil	25 mL
2	onions, sliced	2
2	shallots, chopped	2
2	cloves garlic, minced	2
1	leek (white part only), thinly sliced	1
1 tsp	dried rosemary	5 mL
1	pkg (12 oz/350 g) pizza dough	1
1 cup	freshly grated Parmesan or Asiago cheese (optional, if using)	250 mL

1. Preheat oven to 450°F (230°C). Grease 12-inch (30 cm) pizza pan or spray with nonstick baking spray.

2. In heavy saucepan, heat oil over medium heat; cook onions, shallots, garlic, leek and rosemary, covered, 10 to 12 minutes or until softened.

3. Meanwhile, on floured surface roll out dough to fit prepared pizza pan. Bake for 5 to 8 minutes or until pale brown. Spread onion mixture over dough; continue to bake 20 to 25 minutes or until golden brown on bottom. Remove from oven and sprinkle with cheese (if using). Cut into wedges and serve hot or at room temperature.

Per serving   (1/6th)

Calories	296.3
Protein	12.9 g
Carbohydrate	34.5 g
Fat	11.3 g
Calcium	251.7 mg
	(a high source)
Dietary Fiber	1.6 g

Percent of calories from:

Carbohydrate:	47%
Protein:	18%
Fat:	35%

Roasted Ratatouille Pizza

All the flavors of a classic ratatouille—eggplant, zucchini, peppers, garlic and tomatoes—combine in this roasted version as a pizza topping.

Makes one 12-inch (30 cm) pizza

1	small eggplant, sliced in ½-inch (1 cm) rounds	1
1	small zucchini, sliced	1
Half	red pepper, halved	Half
Half	red onion, sliced	Half
2	cloves garlic, minced	2
8	mushrooms, halved	8
2 tbsp	extra virgin olive oil	25 mL
1	12-inch (30 cm) baked pizza shell	1
1 tbsp	balsamic vinegar	15 mL
1 tsp	each dried basil, rosemary and thyme	5 mL
1 tbsp	freshly grated Parmesan cheese (optional, if tolerated)	15 mL
	Coarse salt and fresh pepper	

1. Preheat broiler. Arrange eggplant, zucchini, red pepper (cup side up), red onion, garlic and mushrooms on baking sheet. Using pastry brush, paint lightly with oil.

2. Broil until browned and lightly charred, 2 to 3 minutes. Remove all vegetables except pepper. Continue broiling red pepper until blackened.

3. Meanwhile, arrange vegetables on pizza shell. Preheat oven to 425°F (220°C).

4. Place charred pepper in plastic container with lid. Let stand 10 minutes. Peel and slice; arrange evenly over pizza.

5. Sprinkle pizza with balsamic vinegar, basil, rosemary, thyme, Parmesan cheese (if using), and salt and pepper to taste.

7. Bake on cookie sheet for 15 to 20 minutes or until heated through. Cut into wedges to serve.

Per serving (1/6th)

Calories	237.5
Protein	6.9 g
Carbohydrate	36.7 g
Fat	6.8 g
Calcium	34.9 mg
Dietary Fiber	3.6 g
	(a source)

Percent of calories from:

Carbohydrate:	62%
Protein:	12%
Fat:	26%

Poultry and Fish

NATURALLY, THERE is no lactose in poultry or fish when it is baked or grilled simply with herbs and a squeeze of lemon. However, these foods lend themselves to magnificent cream-based sauces that cause problems for lactose-intolerant people. The dishes here include basic lactose-reduced sauces rich in flavor to replace their cream-based cousins.

Chicken Without Bother

This is the lazy cook's recipe for preparing succulent, tender chicken in a tasty broth for any of those popular creamy casseroles, pasta dishes and salads or simply to eat on its own. The leftover stock is invaluable for creating a mouth-watering Basic Béchamel Sauce for Chicken Dishes (page 124). Once cooled, the chicken fat can easily be skimmed from the stock. A little chicken fat can then be used for added flavor in the Basic Béchamel Sauce.

1	chicken (3 lb/1.5 kg) or chicken pieces	1
1 cup	chicken stock	250 mL
½ cup	white wine	125 mL
½ tsp	each dried thyme and tarragon	2 mL
1	bay leaf	1

1. Preheat oven to 375°F (190°C). Grease 11- x 7-inch (2 L) baking dish or spray with baking spray.

2. Rinse and pat chicken dry. Arrange in baking dish.

3. In measuring cup, stir together chicken stock, wine, thyme, tarragon and bay leaf; pour over chicken. Cover loosely with foil. Bake for 1-1/2 to 2 hours or until drumsticks wiggle easily and meat thermometer inserted in thickest part of thigh registers 185°F (85°C).

4. When chicken is cool enough to handle, remove meat from carcass; discard bones and skin. Pour remaining chicken stock mixture into container and refrigerate. Chicken fat can be removed from stock once chilled. Cover chicken and refrigerate until ready to use in recipe. Chicken and chicken stock may be frozen for up to 2 months.

Makes about 3 cups (750 mL) chicken and 1 cup (250 mL) chicken stock

Free-range and air-chilled chickens will have more flavor than the more common supermarket variety.

Per serving (1 cup/250 mL)

Calories	477.8
Protein	68.2 g
Carbohydrate	0.9 g
Fat	17.5 g
Calcium	46.3 mg

Percent of calories from:

Carbohydrate:	1%
Protein:	59%
Fat:	34%

Chicken Divan

Makes 4 servings

A comforting dish equally suitable for guests but easy enough for the weekday meal, this can be made up to a day ahead, covered and refrigerated until ready to reheat. Serve with a salad and rice.

1	bunch broccoli	1
3 cups	cooked chicken pieces (see Chicken without Bother, opposite)	750 mL
2 cups	Basic Béchamel Sauce (page 124)	500 mL

Bread Crumb Topping

Recipe doubles easily for serving eight, but requires a 13- x 9-inch (3 L) baking dish.

½ cup	fine dry bread crumbs	125 mL
2 tbsp	extra virgin olive oil	25 mL
2 tbsp	freshly grated Parmesan cheese (optional, if tolerated)	25 mL

1. Preheat oven to 350°F (180°C). Grease 8-inch (2 L) square baking dish.

2. In large saucepan, bring about 1 inch (2.5 cm) water to boil over high heat.

3. Meanwhile, cut off tough part of broccoli stems; slice lengthwise into florets with stem attached. Cook in saucepan of boiling water, uncovered, about 3 minutes or until tender-crisp. Drain and cool.

4. Arrange broccoli in single layer in prepared dish. Arrange chicken over broccoli. Spread Basic Béchamel Sauce over chicken.

5. Bread Crumb Topping: In small bowl, stir together bread crumbs, oil, and cheese (if using) until well blended. Sprinkle evenly over sauce.

6. Bake for 35 to 40 minutes, uncovered, or until heated through and bread crumbs are browned.

Per serving

Calories	390.2
Protein	26.4 g
Carbohydrate	22.8 g
Fat	20.9 g
Calcium	198.8 mg
	(a high source)
Dietary Fiber	3.8 g
	(a source)

Percent of calories from:

Carbohydrate:	23%
Protein:	27%
Fat:	48%

Chicken Pot Pie with Leeks and Mushrooms

This lactose-free treat can be made from soy milk or lactose-reduced milk instead of cream. Serve with Nice 'N' Nutty Slaw (page 52) and crusty bread.

Makes 4 servings

Filling

1 tbsp	chicken fat or vegetable oil	15 mL
2 cups	sliced leeks (2)	500 mL
2 cups	sliced mushrooms	500 mL
2 cups	julienned carrots (3)	500 mL
1 cup	sliced celery	250 mL
½ tsp	dried thyme	2 mL
3 cups	cooked chicken pieces (see Chicken without Bother, page 102)	750 mL
2 cups	Basic Béchamel Sauce (page 124)	500 mL
½ cup	chicken stock	125 mL

Pastry

1 cup	all-purpose flour	250 mL
¼ tsp	salt	1 mL
⅓ cup	shortening	75 mL
3 tbsp	cold water	50 mL

Rolling out pastry is easy with no mess when you put the pastry between 2 sheets of waxed paper and roll away from your body. Roll first in one direction, then turn waxed paper and roll again to make a circular shape.

1. Preheat oven to 425°F (220°C). Grease 8-cup (2 L) baking dish or spray with nonstick baking spray.

2. In large saucepan, melt chicken fat; cook leeks, mushrooms, carrots and celery 4 to 5 minutes or until tender. Stir in thyme, chicken, Basic Béchamel Sauce and stock. Spoon into prepared dish.

3. Pastry: In bowl, stir together flour and salt. Using pastry blender or 2 knives, cut in shortening until in fine crumbs. Stir in water with fork; form into ball. Roll out between 2 sheets of waxed paper and fit on top of chicken mixture. Cut vents in pastry.

4. Bake for 25 to 30 minutes or until pale brown.

Per serving

Calories	577.3
Protein	26.0 g
Carbohydrate	45.0 g
Fat	31.5 g
Calcium	147.8 mg
`	(a source)
Dietary Fiber	5.9 g
	(a high source)

Percent of calories from:

Carbohydrate:	31%
Protein:	18%
Fat:	49%

Turkey Sausages

Makes 4 servings

Commercial sausages and wieners are hidden sources of lactose because skim milk powder is often used as a filler. Not these. If you like sausages, you'll love this lactose-free version. They are low in fat, a snap to make and they taste great!

Serve these in a sesame seed roll with Dijon mustard and pickles.

1 lb	ground turkey	500 g
¼ cup	dry bread crumbs	50 mL
½ tsp	each salt and powdered sage	2 mL
¼ tsp	each grated nutmeg and black pepper	1 mL
1	clove garlic, crushed	1

1. In mixing bowl, combine turkey, bread crumbs, salt, sage, nutmeg, pepper and garlic, until evenly distributed. Shape into wiener, meatball or patty shapes.

2. Cook over medium-high in nonstick skillet for about 15 minutes, turning, until brown on all sides and cooked through.

Per serving

Calories	166.9
Protein	15.8 g
Carbohydrate	5.0 g
Fat	8.8 g
Calcium	28.5 mg
Dietary Fiber	0.3 g

Percent of calories from:
Carbohydrate:	12%
Protein:	39%
Fat:	49%

Herb-Roasted Turkey

Once you have prepared your turkey using this no-fuss method on the barbecue, you are a convert for life! It cooks in double-quick time and leaves your oven free for all the vegetable casseroles, too.

Makes about 12 servings

Do not use a pre-basted turkey for this method. The added oil will flare up on the barbecue.

1	fresh turkey	1
	12 to 16 lb (5.5 to 7.25 kg)	
1	onion	1
1	celery stick	1
2 tbsp	each fresh lemon juice and olive oil	25 mL
2 tsp	dried thyme	10 mL
½ tsp	dried rosemary	2 mL

1. Preheat barbecue to medium-high. Spread liquid dishwasher detergent on outside of roasting pan for easy clean up or use disposable foil pan.

2. Remove neck and giblets from turkey. Rinse under cold water and pat dry with paper towels. Tuck wings under back. Place on rack in pan.

3. Place onion and celery in cavity. Squeeze lemon juice on outside of bird. Sprinkle evenly with oil, thyme and rosemary. Pour 2 to 3 cups (500 mL to 750 mL) water into pan. Cover bird with two layers of foil.

4. Place on barbecue grill; close lid. Cook for 2 to 2-1/2 hours, replenishing water if necessary, or until meat thermometer registers 170°F (77°C). Remove from pan and let stand, covered, for 15 minutes before carving.

Per serving

Calories	646.2
Protein	104.8 g
Carbohydrate	1.9 g
Fat	21.4 g
Calcium	102.5 mg
	(a source)
Dietary Fiber	0.4 g

Percent of calories from:

Carbohydrate:	1%
Protein:	68%
Fat:	31%

Loaf Pan Carrot Stuffing

Makes 1 loaf (8 servings)

To toast almonds, spread on baking sheet and bake in preheated 350°F (180°C) oven 10 to 15 minutes or until golden brown and fragrant.
   The dry ingredients for the stuffing may be assembled the night before, ready for the liquid ingredients to be added at the last minute.

Baking a stuffing separately makes for a lighter, more easily digested dressing without absorbing the fat from the turkey. Of course, it is easier to serve! This is a family favorite that's been modified using shortening and orange juice instead of my usual butter and milk. Almonds are added for calcium.

1 cup	all-purpose flour	250 mL
1 cup	fresh bread crumbs	250 mL
1	carrot, coarsely grated (1 cup/250 mL)	1
½ cup	toasted chopped unblanched almonds	125 mL
1 tsp	baking powder	5 mL
½ tsp	each salt, ground ginger and nutmeg	2 mL
¼ cup	each vegetable oil and packed brown sugar	50 mL
1	egg	1
⅓ cup	orange juice	75 mL

1. Preheat oven to 350°F (180°C). Grease 9- x 5-inch (2 L) loaf pan.

2. In mixing bowl, stir together flour, bread crumbs, carrot, almonds, baking powder, salt, ginger and nutmeg.

3. In separate bowl, beat together oil and sugar until fluffy; beat in egg and orange juice. Stir into dry ingredients just until moistened. Spoon into prepared pan.

4. Cover pan with foil. Bake for 50 to 60 minutes or until firm to touch and toothpick inserted in center comes away clean.

Per serving

Calories	343.4
Protein	8.5 g
Carbohydrate	41.6 g
Fat	16.9 g
Calcium	93.4 mg
	(a source)
Dietary Fiber	3.7 g
	(a source)

Percent of calories from:

Carbohydrate:	47%
Protein:	10%
Fat:	43%

Salmon Mousse

My adaptation of my mother's delicious recipe is lactose-free, but screams of cream! Serve it with Cucumber Almond Salad (page 61) and bread, and garnish with sliced cucumber and lemon.

Makes 4 cups (1 L) or 6 servings

1	pkg (10.25 oz/290 g) silken soft tofu	1
1½	pkg gelatin (4½ tsp/22 mL)	1½
3 tbsp	fresh lemon juice	50 mL
½ cup	boiling water	125 mL
2	cans (each 7.5 oz/213 g) salmon	2
½ cup	light salad dressing	125 mL
¼ cup	each chopped fresh dill and green onion	50 mL
¼ tsp	black pepper	1 mL

1. Using sieve, drain tofu. Line 4-cup (1 L) mold or small loaf pan with plastic wrap.

2. In small mixing bowl, sprinkle gelatin over lemon juice. Let stand about 5 minutes or until lemon juice has been absorbed. Stir in boiling water until gelatin is dissolved.

3. Drain salmon, discarding skin and reserving bones. In food processor, combine salmon and bones, tofu, salad dressing, dill, onion and pepper; purée until smooth. With motor running, pour dissolved gelatin through feed tube.

4. Spoon salmon mixture into prepared pan; cover and refrigerate about 2 hours or until firm. May be made the night before. To unmold, place serving platter over mold; invert mold and, using plastic wrap as lever, gently ease mousse onto platter. Remove plastic wrap. Slice into 1/2-inch (1 cm) pieces.

Per serving
(2/3 cup/150 mL)

Calories	212
Protein	16.2 g
Carbohydrate	4.9 g
Fat	13.9 g
Calcium	183.1 mg
	(a high source)
Dietary Fiber	0.1 g

Percent of calories from:

Carbohydrate:	9%
Protein:	31%
Fat:	60%

Fish Fingers

Makes 4 servings

Breading for fish and chicken in the popular frozen food section of the supermarket is a hidden source of lactose (milk powder in the bread crumbs), which can cause problems for those with lactose-intolerance. This recipe makes everyone happy. It's delicious with Green Sauce (page 128).

Chicken Fingers: Substitute fresh chicken strips for fish and bake at 375°F (190°C) 30 to 35 minutes or until no longer pink inside.

1	pkg (400 g) individually frozen fish fillets (sole, haddock or cod), thawed or use fresh	1
1 tbsp	vegetable oil	15 mL

Breading

½ cup	dry bread crumbs	125 mL
¼ tsp	each salt, paprika, dried thyme, granulated sugar and pepper	1 mL
2 tbsp	vegetable oil	25 mL

The method for fresh fillets is different from frozen fillets because bread crumbs will stick to fresh but not frozen fillets.

1. Preheat oven to 450°F (230°C). Grease 13- x 9-inch (3 L) baking dish.

2. Breading: In mixing bowl, stir together bread crumbs, salt, paprika, thyme, sugar and pepper. Stir in oil.

3. Cut each fillet in half lengthwise to make a long, fat "finger."

4. If using frozen fillets, brush with oil; arrange in single layer in prepared dish and sprinkle breading evenly over fillets. If using fresh fillets, brush lightly with oil; dip into bread crumbs to coat on each side. Arrange in single layer in baking dish.

5. Bake for 10 to 15 minutes or until fish flakes easily when tested with fork.

Per serving

Calories	221.6
Protein	18.3 g
Carbohydrate	9.6 g
Fat	11.9 g
Calcium	31.0 mg
Dietary Fiber	0.5 g

Percent of calories from:

Carbohydrate:	18%
Protein:	33%
Fat:	49%

Fisherman's Pie

Children are guaranteed to like this soothing dish, a mashed potato crust with a well-seasoned filling.

Makes 4 servings

Potato Shell

6	medium potatoes, peeled (about 2¼ lb/1 kg)	6
1 cup	lactose-reduced milk or soy milk	250 mL
½ tsp	salt	2 mL
Pinch	each nutmeg and black pepper	Pinch

Coquilles St. Jacques: Substitute fresh sea scallops for fish. In Step 4, reduce cooking time to 3 minutes or just until scallops are opaque.

Fish Filling

1½ cups	water	375 mL
½ cup	dry white wine	125 mL
1	bay leaf	1
1	each carrot and celery, coarsely chopped	1
1	onion	1
4	whole cloves	4
1 lb	sole or haddock, fresh or frozen	500 g
1 tbsp	vegetable oil	15 mL
1 cup	each sliced mushrooms and leeks	250 mL
2 tbsp	all-purpose flour	25 mL

1. Spray 10-inch (1.5 L) pie plate with nonstick baking spray.

2. Potato Shell: In saucepan, cover potatoes with cold water and bring to boil; reduce heat and simmer until tender, 20 to 25 minutes. Drain and mash with fork or potato masher. Beat in milk, salt, nutmeg and pepper until fluffy. Spread over bottom and sides of prepared pie plate, making decorative swirls.

Per serving

Calories	433.5
Protein	26.9 g
Carbohydrate	63.5 g
Fat	6.4 g
Calcium	137.6 mg (a source)
Dietary Fiber	7.1 g (a very high source)

Percent of calories from:

Carbohydrate:	58%
Protein:	25%
Fat:	13%

3. Fish Filling: Meanwhile, in saucepan, bring water, wine, bay leaf, carrot, celery and onion stuck with whole cloves to boil. Simmer about 15 minutes.

4. Arrange fish in saucepan, cutting into large chunks if necessary to fit pan. Bring to boil. Reduce heat and simmer until fish flakes easily when tested with fork, 5 to 10 minutes depending on whether fish was fresh or frozen. Drain and reserve stock and fish. Discard vegetables and bay leaf.

5. Preheat oven to 425°F (220°C).

6. In saucepan, heat oil over medium heat; cook mushrooms and leeks until tender, about 5 minutes. Sprinkle with flour; stir until smooth. Remove from heat. Gradually whisk in reserved fish stock. Return to heat. Cook, stirring, until thickened, about 2 minutes. Stir in reserved fish. Taste and adjust seasonings.

7. Spoon filling into potato shell. Bake for 20 to 25 minutes or until golden brown around edges. Cut into wedges to serve.

Grilled Salmon

Preparing salmon for oven grilling or barbecuing takes minutes, and the dish doesn't require a buttery basting during cooking. A mere squeeze of lemon is all that is required to complete this salmon perfection.

Makes 1 serving

4 oz	salmon fillet	125 g
1 tbsp	white wine	15 mL
1½ tsp	extra virgin olive oil	7 mL
2 tsp	chopped fresh tarragon or dill	10 mL
	Black pepper	

1. Preheat oven to 450°F (230°C) or barbecue to medium-high. Spray baking pan with nonstick baking spray or if using barbecue, spray a piece of foil.

2. Arrange salmon fillet skin side down, in prepared dish or foil. Sprinkle with wine, olive oil, tarragon and pepper.

3. Bake or grill 10 to 15 minutes, depending on thickness of fillet, until fish is opaque and flakes easily when tested with fork.

Per serving

Calories	176.1
Protein	16.4 g
Carbohydrate	0.6 g
Fat	10.6 g
Calcium	21.9 mg
Dietary Fiber	0.0 g

Percent of calories from:

Carbohydrate:	1%
Protein:	38%
Fat:	55%

Vegetables

WHO DOESN'T love that wonderful comfort food, mashed
potatoes, or, for that matter, scalloped potatoes?
This section provides recipes for these popular creamy
vegetable dishes. In addition, it includes vegetable
dishes containing available calcium, that is calcium
that can be absorbed by our bodies. There are a
number of vegetables with this mineral but only
some of them have available calcium. See chart
page 12.

Quick Sauté of Collard Greens

Collards are the oldest of all relations to the cabbage and a vegetable source of available calcium. They have a wonderful tangy taste that complements ham, pork and stew recipes. The large, dark green, paddle-shaped leaves need to have their tough stem removed before being boiled in water. Afterwards, they may be sautéed, as in this recipe, or combined in a béchamel sauce as an accompaniment dish.

1	bunch collard greens (12 oz/375 g)	1
1 tbsp	extra virgin olive oil	15 mL
1	clove garlic, crushed	1

1. Remove tough central collard stem. Boil uncovered in large pot of water about 15 minutes.

2. Drain well. Chop coarsely.

3. Heat olive oil in saucepan over medium heat. Add garlic and collards, stir-frying about 2 minutes to heat through and coat lightly with oil-garlic mixture. Serve at once.

Makes 4 servings

Per serving
(nutrient analysis shown for turnip greens, which are similar)

Calories	48.2
Protein	1.0 g
Carbohydrate	4.0 g
Fat	3.6 g
Calcium	117.7 mg
	(a source)
Dietary Fiber	2.6 g
	(a source)

Percent of calories from:

Carbohydrate:	30%
Protein:	8%
Fat:	62%

Stir Fry of Greens

Makes 4 servings

Ready in minutes, this calcium-containing stir fry is a delectable side dish or a quick vegetarian main course with the addition of crumbled tofu. Serve over basmati rice.

1	bunch bok choy (12 oz/375g)	1
1	broccoli stalk (⅓ bunch)	1
1	stalk celery	1
Half	green pepper, sliced	Half
1 cup	sliced mushrooms (4 oz/125 g)	250 mL
2 tbsp	vegetable oil	25 mL
1	clove garlic, crushed	1
½ cup	water	125 mL
¼ cup	soy sauce	50 mL
1 tsp	sesame oil	5 mL
2 tbsp	sesame seeds	25 mL

1. Slice bok choy into 1/2-inch (1 cm) pieces; cut broccoli into florets and slice the tender part of stem; slice celery on the diagonal. Combine with sliced green pepper and mushrooms and set aside.

2. In wok or large saucepan, heat vegetable oil over medium-high and stir-fry garlic about 30 seconds. Add vegetables, stirring to coat. Add water and cook about 5 minutes until tender-crisp.

3. Stir in soy sauce and sesame oil. Serve immediately with a sprinkle of sesame seeds.

Per serving

Calories	142.8
Protein	5.0 g
Carbohydrate	9.7 g
Fat	10.4 g
Calcium	154.2 mg
	(a source)
Dietary Fiber	4.0 g
	(a high source)

Percent of calories from:

Carbohydrate:	25%
Protein:	13%
Fat:	62%

Braised Kale

Calcium-rich kale, a member of the cabbage family, has a piquant flavor and coarse texture, which lends itself to this simple but tasty recipe—a wonderful accompaniment to roast pork.

Makes 4 servings

1	bunch kale, washed	1
2 tbsp	extra virgin olive oil	25 mL
1	clove garlic, crushed	1
	Salt and pepper	

1. Remove tough stems from kale. In large saucepan, bring about 1/2 inch (1 cm) water to boil; add kale. Return to boil; simmer, covered, for 3 to 4 minutes or until limp. Drain well. Chop coarsely.

2. In same saucepan, heat oil over medium heat; cook garlic about 1 minute or until softened. Add kale; cook, stirring, for 1 minute until heated through. Season to taste with salt and pepper. Serve immediately.

Per serving

Calories	526.9
Protein	3.2 g
Carbohydrate	8.6 g
Fat	54.2 g
Calcium	203.0 mg
	(a high source)
Dietary Fiber	0.7 g

Percent of calories from:
Carbohydrate:	6%
Protein:	2%
Fat:	91%

Mashed Potato Casserole

Makes 8 to 10 servings

Don't try to short circuit this recipe by using the food processor to mash potatoes: you will have glue before you know it. Mash with a potato masher or electric mixer.

Humble mashed potatoes have become chic food these days with added sautéed garlic to give zing. And for many people, the simple mashed potato of their childhood is a must to accompany Christmas dinner. Feel free to halve this recipe for a smaller quantity. If you want enough for leftovers, beat in a little more milk the next day to keep them at their creamy best. You can prepare this make-ahead casserole up to two days before serving.

5 lb	baking potatoes	2.2 kg
2 cups	2% lactose-reduced milk	500 mL
1 tsp	salt	5 mL
½ tsp	each black pepper and nutmeg	2 mL

1. Preheat oven to 350°F (180°C). Grease 13- x 9-inch (3 L) baking dish.

2. Peel and quarter potatoes. In large saucepan, cover potatoes with cold water and bring to boil. Reduce heat and simmer, covered, 20 to 25 minutes or until very tender. Drain well.

3. Using electric mixer or potato masher, mash potatoes until smooth. Beat in milk, salt, pepper and nutmeg.

4. Spoon into prepared baking dish; cover with foil. Casserole can be refrigerated for up to 2 days. Bake for 45 to 60 minutes or until piping hot.

Per serving (1/8th)

Calories	299.7
Protein	7.6 g
Carbohydrate	64.1 g
Fat	2.1 g
Calcium	90.9 mg
	(a source)
Dietary Fiber	6.1 g
	(a very high source)

Percent of calories from:

Carbohydrate:	84%
Protein:	10%
Fat:	6%

Carrot Squash Crumble

This oh-so-good casserole is almost like dessert. The crunchy nutty topping is an interesting contrast to the smooth interior of this make-ahead dish. For added speed, use frozen chopped squash, which requires no preparation and only minutes of cooking.

Makes 8 to 10 servings

2 lb	butternut squash	1 kg
2 lb	carrots	1 kg
¾ cup	orange juice	175 mL
2 tbsp	packed brown sugar	25 mL
1 tsp	each salt and cinnamon	5 mL

Nutty Topping

1¼ cups	fresh bread crumbs	300 mL
½ cup	toasted almonds, chopped	125 mL
2 tbsp	olive oil	25 mL
½ tsp	salt	2 mL

1. Preheat oven to 350°F (180°C). Grease 13- x 9-inch (3 L) baking dish.

2. Peel and coarsely chop squash and carrots. In large pot of boiling water, cook carrots and fresh squash until very tender, 25 to 30 minutes. If using frozen squash, add to carrots for last 15 minutes of cooking. Drain thoroughly.

3. Using food processor or potato masher, purée vegetables until smooth. Beat in orange juice, sugar, salt and cinnamon. Spoon into prepared casserole.

4. Nutty Topping: In mixing bowl, combine bread crumbs, almonds, oil and salt; sprinkle over casserole. Crumble can be covered and refrigerated for up to 2 days. Bake, uncovered, for 50 to 60 minutes or until piping hot.

Per serving (1/8th)

Calories	242.8
Protein	6.3 g
Carbohydrate	42.6 g
Fat	7.2 g
Calcium	136.4 mg
	(a source)
Dietary Fiber	6.5 g
	(a very high source)

Percent of calories from:

Carbohydrate:	65%
Protein:	10%
Fat:	25%

Scalloped Potatoes

Makes 8 servings

Yukon Gold and baking potatoes make the best scalloped potatoes.

You can never have too much scalloped potatoes, so allow two potatoes per person. If there are any leftovers, they are a welcome addition to dinner the next night. This foolproof method ensures lots of creamy sauce to coat potatoes.

5 lb	potatoes, peeled and halved	2.2 kg
¼ cup	all-purpose flour	50 mL
2 tbsp	vegetable oil	25 mL
6 cups	lactose-reduced milk or soy milk	1.5 L
1 tsp	salt	5 mL
¼ tsp	each black pepper and nutmeg	1 mL

Topping

½ cup	fine dry bread crumbs	125 mL
2 tbsp	extra virgin olive oil	25 mL
2 tbsp	freshly grated Parmesan cheese (if tolerated)	25 mL

1. In large saucepan, cover potatoes with cold water; bring to boil. Reduce heat and simmer until barely tender, 12 to 15 minutes. Drain well and let cool; slice thickly.

2. In same saucepan, stir together flour and oil until smooth; cook over medium heat until starting to pull away from bottom of pan. Remove from heat. Gradually whisk in milk until smooth. Return to medium heat; cook, whisking frequently, until thickened. Whisk in salt, pepper and nutmeg.

3. Preheat oven to 350°F (180°C). Grease 13- x 9-inch (3 L) baking dish. Spoon in potatoes; pour sauce over top.

4. Topping: In mixing bowl, stir together bread crumbs, oil and cheese until well mixed. Sprinkle evenly over potatoes. Bake for 30 to 35 minutes or until heated through.

Per serving

Calories	425.3
Protein	12.6 g
Carbohydrate	72.1 g
Fat	10.3 g
Calcium	275.7 mg
	(a very high source)
Dietary Fiber	5.8 g
	(a high source)

Percent of calories from:

Carbohydrate:	67%
Protein:	12%
Fat:	21%

Carrots with Maple Syrup

A variation on glazed carrots, this version without butter is the perfect companion to the Easter menu.

2 lb	carrots, peeled	1 kg
¼ cup	pure maple syrup	50 mL
	Salt and pepper to taste	

1. Using sharp knife, cut carrots into julienne strips, 4- x 1/4-inch (10 cm x 5 mm).

2. In large saucepan or Dutch oven, bring 1-1/2 cups (375 mL) water to boil. Add carrots and return to boil; simmer, covered, 3 to 4 minutes or until crisp-tender. Drain.

3. Pour in maple syrup stirring gently to combine. Return to boil and boil, uncovered, until thickened slightly, 2 to 3 minutes. Serve immediately.

Per serving

Calories	138.5
Protein	2.3 g
Carbohydrate	33.6 g
Fat	0.4 g
Calcium	79.2 mg
	(a source)
Dietary Fiber	5.5 g
	(a high source)

Percent of calories from:

Carbohydrate:	91%
Protein:	6%
Fat:	3%

Artichokes with Spicy Lemon Sauce

Makes 4 servings

Artichokes make a wonderful starter before a fish or seafood main course, especially in spring when they are plentiful.

To eat these delectable morsels, pull off leaves one at a time; dip into sauce and drag the leaf through your teeth to remove the tender, delicate "meat" of the artichoke.

Per serving

Calories	169.7
Protein	4.6 g
Carbohydrate	15.6 g
Fat	11.7 g
Calcium	68.0 mg
	(a source)
Dietary Fiber	4.1 g
	(a high source)

Percent of calories from:

Carbohydrate:	33%
Protein:	10%
Fat:	57%

This is a favorite appetizer I make all the time with a spicy lemon butter mixture as a dipping sauce. However, for the cookbook, I came up with this lactose-free version using olive oil to replace the rich taste of butter—with great success! All preparation can be done ahead, then just a few last-minute touches are necessary. Try to find artichokes of a similar size.

4	medium artichokes	4

Spicy Lemon Sauce

⅓ cup	fresh lemon juice	75 mL
¼ cup	extra virgin olive oil	50 mL
2	cloves garlic, crushed	2
1 tsp	each Worcestershire sauce, dried tarragon and salt	5 mL
¼ tsp	black pepper	1 mL
Pinch	cayenne pepper	Pinch

1. Using sharp knife, cut 1/2 inch (1 cm) off stem end and tips of leaves.

2. In steamer over simmering water, steam artichokes for 35 to 40 minutes or until very tender. May be prepared several hours ahead, then reheated just before serving.

3. Spicy Lemon Sauce: In saucepan, bring lemon juice, oil, garlic, Worcestershire sauce, tarragon, salt, pepper and cayenne to boil; reduce heat and simmer for 1 minute. Sauce may be prepared up to 1 hour ahead, then returned to boil just before serving.

4. To serve, arrange artichokes in individual serving bowls. Spoon about 2 tbsp (25 mL) hot sauce over each serving of artichokes. Serve at once.

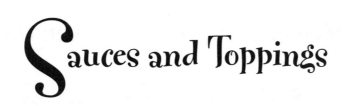

Sauces and Toppings

Basic Béchamel Sauce for Chicken Dishes

This lactose-free version of béchamel sauce has a velvety texture and rich flavor—the perfect complement to any chicken casserole calling for a cream or béchamel sauce.

Makes 4 servings

3 tbsp	all-purpose flour	50 mL
2 tbsp	vegetable oil or chicken fat	25 mL
1 cup	chicken stock	250 mL
1	bay leaf	1
¼ cup	white wine or sherry	50 mL
1 cup	lactose-reduced milk or soy milk	250 mL
	Salt and black pepper	

1. In saucepan, stir together flour and oil until smooth. Heat over medium-high heat until bubbly. Remove from heat.

2. Gradually whisk in chicken stock and bay leaf. Return to heat. Cook, stirring, over medium heat for 4 to 5 minutes or until thickened and smooth.

3. Stir in wine; cook 1 minute. Gradually whisk in milk; cook over medium-high heat, stirring, about 5 minutes. Discard bay leaf. Season to taste with salt and pepper.

Variation:

Mushroom Cream Sauce: Cook 1-1/2 cups (375 mL) sliced mushrooms in vegetable oil until liquid is released, about 5 minutes. Sprinkle with flour and stir until smooth. Continue with recipe.

Per serving
(1/2 cup/125 mL)

Calories	132
Protein	3.9 g
Carbohydrate	7.8 g
Fat	8.4 g
Calcium	79.9 mg
Dietary Fiber	0.2 g

Percent of calories from:

Carbohydrate:	24%
Protein:	12%
Fat:	57%

Gremolata Bread Crumbs

Makes about 2½ cups
(625 mL)

The flavors of Provence combine in this zesty mixture that's ideal for a coating or stuffing for fish, seafood, poultry, veal and a topping for pasta.

Seasoned bread crumbs are a great flavor substitute for many recipes where cheese or cream sauces play a major role. Commercial bread crumb coatings may contain lactose in the form of milk solids. (Check the list of ingredients on package label.) Making your own bread crumbs without lactose is easy. Simply break up a piece of bread and process in the blender or food processor. For variety, use whole wheat, rye or mixed-grain breads.

2 cups	fresh bread crumbs (from Italian or French bread)	500 mL
½ cup	chopped fresh parsley	125 mL
2 tbsp	grated lemon rind	25 mL
1 tbsp	freshly grated Parmesan cheese (optional, if tolerated)	15 mL
1 tbsp	extra virgin olive oil	15 mL
1 tsp	dried tarragon	5 mL
½ tsp	each salt and dried basil	2 mL
¼ tsp	black pepper	1 mL

1. In mixing bowl, combine bread crumbs, parsley, lemon rind, cheese (if using), oil, tarragon, salt, basil and pepper. Taste and adjust seasonings.

2. May be refrigerated in airtight container for up to 2 days or frozen for up to 2 months.

Per serving
(1/2 cup/125 mL)

Calories	190.9
Protein	6.0 g
Carbohydrate	30.4 g
Fat	5.2 g
Calcium	86.1 mg
	(a source)
Dietary Fiber	1.8 g

Percent of calories from:
Carbohydrate:	63%
Protein:	12%
Fat:	24%

Rosemary Sun-Dried Tomato Crumb Topping

Use this robust-flavored crumb topping for pasta dishes such as lasagne, or as a coating or stuffing for meat or poultry.

Makes about 1⅓ cups (325 mL)

1 cup	fresh bread crumbs (from Italian or French bread)	250 mL
¼ cup	chopped fresh parsley	50 mL
2 tbsp	diced sun-dried tomato packed in oil	25 mL
1 tbsp	freshly grated Parmesan cheese (optional, if tolerated)	15 mL
1 tbsp	extra virgin olive oil	15 mL
½ tsp	dried basil	2 mL
Pinch	each dried rosemary and black pepper	Pinch

1. In mixing bowl, combine bread crumbs, parsley, tomato, cheese (if using), olive oil, basil, rosemary and pepper. Taste and adjust seasonings.

2. May be refrigerated in airtight container for up to 2 days or frozen for up to 2 months.

Sun-dried tomatoes can be purchased dried in a package or in oil in a jar. The oil-packed ones are more expensive. To reconstitute dry-packed tomatoes, place in a saucepan and cover with hot water; add a bay leaf and bring to boil. Reduce heat and simmer until tomatoes are tender, 5 to 10 minutes; drain. May be used at this point but for more flavor, place in a jar; cover with extra virgin olive oil and crushed garlic and basil or fennel if you wish. Refrigerate for up to 2 weeks.

Per serving   1/3 cup (75mL)

Calories	147.2
Protein	4.5 g
Carbohydrate	20.7 g
Fat	5.5 g
Calcium	79.8 mg
Dietary Fiber	1.7 g

Percent of calories from:

Carbohydrate:	55%
Protein:	12%
Fat:	33%

Tofu "Sour Cream" for Baked Potatoes

Makes about 1¼ cups
(300 mL)

To serve with baked
potatoes, bake scrubbed
potatoes in preheated 425°F
(220°C) oven about 1 hour or
until tender. Using sharp
knife, cut X into potato and
top with a dollop of Tofu
"Sour Cream."

You don't need to feel deprived when you serve this tofu cream on your baked potatoes or with any food such as tortilla chips and crudités where you would normally want some sour cream.

1	pkg (10.25 oz/290 g) silken firm tofu	1
1 tbsp	each fresh lemon juice and vegetable oil	15 mL
½ tsp	each salt and granulated sugar	2 mL

Zesty Toppers (optional)

¼ cup	each chopped sweet red pepper and jalapeño pepper	50 mL
2 tbsp	chopped black olives	25 mL

1. Using sieve, drain tofu.

2. In food processor, purée together drained tofu, lemon juice, oil, salt and sugar until smooth.

3. Zesty Toppers: For added zest, stir in red pepper, jalapeño pepper and olives.

4. Cover and refrigerate for up to 2 days.

Per serving   (2 tbsp/25 mL)

Plain Tofu Cream:

Calories	25.6
Protein	1.6 g
Carbohydrate	0.9 g
Fat	1.8 g
Calcium	7.5 mg
Dietary Fiber	0.0 g

Percent of calories from:

Carbohydrate:	13%
Protein:	25%
Fat:	62%

Green Sauce

This is my favorite all-purpose sauce to be served with any fish, especially salmon. It works well as a dip for vegetables too!

Makes 1 cup (250 mL)

1	pkg (10.25 oz/290 g) silken soft tofu	1
¼ cup	each chopped fresh dill, parsley and green onions	50 mL
2 tbsp	each fresh lemon juice and light mayonnaise	25 mL
½ tsp	salt	2 mL
¼ tsp	black pepper	1 mL

1. Using sieve, drain tofu.

2. In food processor, purée drained tofu, dill, parsley, onions, lemon juice, mayonnaise, salt and pepper until smooth.

3. Spoon into container; cover and refrigerate up to 3 days.

Per serving (2 tbsp/25 mL)

Calories	41.0
Protein	1.9 g
Carbohydrate	2.3 g
Fat	2.9 g
Calcium	23.9 mg
Dietary Fiber	0.1 g

Percent of calories from:

Carbohydrate:	21%
Protein:	18%
Fat:	61%

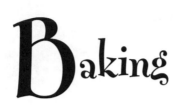

Baking

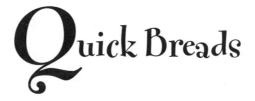

Quick Breads

BREADS AND other baking often rely on milk and butter because they have unique qualities which provide flavor, browning and sweetness. Milk also reacts with the leavening agents to make baked products rise nicely and stay risen. Baking without milk proved quite a challenge!

We discovered fruit purées, fruit juice, coffee, beer, lactose-reduced milk and soy milk gave moisture. As we tested, we found a bonus—the fruit purées and fruit not only provided liquid but also meant we were often able to reduce fat content compared to the original recipe.

We had many failures as we worked to create delicious results. They had to taste so scrumptious that you will want to start baking all your own breads!

Whole Grain Seed and Nut Bread

Make this bread in minutes and enjoy the results sliced and toasted with marmalade or fresh for an accompaniment to soup and salad. The bread will keep refrigerated for up to five days or frozen for up to three months.

Makes a 9-inch (2 L) loaf

Make the bread in small loaf pans for gifts or for cocktail bread but reduce the baking time. Start checking bread at 30 minutes for doneness. It is excellent served with Salmon Mousse (page 108)

2 cups	all-purpose flour	500 mL
1 cup	each whole wheat flour, quick-cooking rolled oats and natural bran	250 mL
½ cup	toasted chopped almonds or hazelnuts	125 mL
2 tbsp	each sesame seeds, poppyseeds and pumpkin seeds	25 mL
2 tsp	baking powder	10 mL
1 tsp	each baking soda and salt	5 mL
1½ cups	soy milk or lactose-reduced milk	375 mL
⅓ cup	liquid honey	75 mL

To toast nuts, spread on cookie sheet and bake in preheated 350°F (180°C) oven 12 to 15 minutes or until fragrant.

1. Preheat oven to 350°F (180°C). Line 9- x 5-inch (2 L) loaf pan with waxed paper.

2. In mixing bowl, stir together all-purpose flour, whole wheat flour, rolled oats, bran, almonds, sesame seeds, poppyseeds, pumpkin seeds, baking powder, baking soda and salt. Stir in milk and honey just until dry ingredients are moistened.

3. Spoon batter into prepared pan. Bake for about 1 hour or until toothpick inserted in center comes away clean. Cool before cutting into slices. May be well wrapped and frozen for up to 3 months.

Per serving (1/2 inch/1 cm)

Calories	153.7
Protein	5.4 g
Carbohydrate	27.3 g
Fat	3.6 g
Calcium	49.8 mg
Dietary Fiber	3.0 g
	(a source)

Percent of calories from:

Carbohydrate:	67%
Protein:	13%
Fat:	20%

Beer Bread

Makes a 9-inch (2 L) loaf

Beer gives this bread a yeasty flavor and an unusual zing! It is an excellent companion to hearty soups such as Mushroom Chowder (page 46).

2 cups	all-purpose flour	500 mL
1 cup	whole wheat flour	250 mL
¼ cup	loosely packed brown sugar	50 mL
1 tbsp	baking powder	15 mL
2 tsp	caraway or dill seeds	10 mL
1 tsp	salt	5 mL
1	bottle (341 mL) beer	1
1 tbsp	caraway or dill seeds (optional)	15 mL

1. Preheat oven to 350°F (180°C). Line 9- x 5-inch (2 L) loaf pan with waxed paper.

2. In mixing bowl, stir together all-purpose flour, whole wheat flour, sugar, baking powder, caraway seeds and salt. Stir in beer just until dry ingredients are moistened.

3. Spoon batter into prepared pan. Sprinkle with more seeds for garnish if desired.

4. Bake for 55 to 60 minutes or until toothpick inserted in center comes out clean. Let cool before slicing.

Per serving (1/2 inch/1 cm)

Calories	92.8
Protein	2.5 g
Carbohydrate	18.7 g
Fat	0.3 g
Calcium	17.8 mg
Dietary Fiber	1.4 g

Percent of calories from:

Carbohydrate:	80%
Protein:	11%
Fat:	3%

Double Cornbread

A moist bread with the rich sweetness of corn, this is ideal to pack for lunch or serve with soup or salad.

Makes 1 round cake or 10 large muffins

1 cup	cake-and-pastry flour	250 mL
1 cup	cornmeal	250 mL
2 tsp	baking powder	10 mL
1 tsp	baking soda	5 mL
½ tsp	salt	2 mL
½ cup	shortening	125 mL
¼ cup	granulated sugar	50 mL
1	egg	1
1 cup	creamed corn	250 mL
½ cup	water	125 mL
	Sesame seeds	

To cut cornbread cake, loosen edges with knife, invert onto wire rack and remove waxed paper. Place serving plate on cake and invert onto serving plate. Cut into wedges.

1. Preheat oven to 375°F (190°C). Line bottom of 9-inch (1.5 L) round cake pan with waxed paper or line 10 large muffin tins with paper baking cups.

2. In mixing bowl, stir together flour, cornmeal, baking powder, baking soda and salt.

3. In separate bowl and using electric mixer, beat together shortening and sugar until fluffy. Beat in egg, creamed corn and water until well combined. Stir into dry ingredients just until moistened.

4. Spoon into prepared pan or muffin cups. Sprinkle with sesame seeds.

5. Bake muffins for 20 to 25 minutes, cake for 30 to 35 minutes or until firm to touch or toothpick inserted in center comes out clean. Let stand for about 15 minutes before removing paper.

6. Bread can be covered and refrigerated for up to 2 days, or wrapped well and frozen for up to 3 months.

Creamed corn replaces the milk in this recipe to give the necessary moisture.

Per serving   (1/2 inch/1 cm)

Calories	129.4
Protein	1.9 g
Carbohydrate	16.0 g
Fat	6.6 g
Calcium	15.8 mg
Dietary Fiber	0.9 g

Percent of calories from:

Carbohydrate:	49%
Protein:	6%
Fat:	45%

Caraway Currant Soda Bread

Makes a 9-inch (23 cm) circular loaf

Dazzle your friends with this quickly made bread. It's great served hot from the oven cut into wedges or sliced and spread with Pear Butter (page 164).

Soaking currants cleans and plumps them up, making them juicier in recipes.

¾ cup	currants	175 mL
3 cups	whole wheat flour	750 mL
1 cup	all-purpose flour	250 mL
2 tsp	baking powder	10 mL
1 tsp	each baking soda and salt	5 mL
1½ cups	water	375 mL
¼ cup	each liquid honey and vegetable oil	50 mL
2 tsp	caraway seeds	10 mL
	Granulated sugar	

1. Preheat oven to 350°F (180°C). In small bowl, soak currants in warm water. Grease baking sheet.

2. In mixing bowl, stir together whole wheat flour, all-purpose flour, baking powder, baking soda and salt. Drain currants and add to bowl. Stir in water, honey, oil and caraway seeds just until dry ingredients are moistened.

3. Knead with floured hands until smooth, about 1 minute. Shape into 7-inch (18 cm) circle. Place on prepared baking sheet. Cut large X about 1/4 inch (5 mm) deep on top; sprinkle with sugar.

4. Bake for about 1 hour or until toothpick inserted in center comes out clean.

Per serving (1/8th)

Calories	299.3
Protein	8.0 g
Carbohydrate	54.6 g
Fat	6.9 g
Calcium	38.9 mg
Dietary Fiber	6.6 g
(a very high source)	

Percent of calories from:

Carbohydrate:	70%
Protein:	10%
Fat:	20%

Blueberry Cornbread

Make the most of fresh blueberries in this luscious breakfast or teatime treat. For more blueberry flavor, serve with Quick Blueberry Sauce (variation page 208).

Makes a 9-inch (2 L) loaf

1½ cups	all-purpose flour	375 mL
1 cup	cornmeal	250 mL
¾ cup	granulated sugar	175 mL
2 tsp	each grated lemon and orange rind	10 mL
1 tsp	baking soda	5 mL
½ tsp	salt	2 mL
2	eggs	2
½ cup	orange juice	125 mL
¼ cup	vegetable oil	50 mL
1½ cups	fresh blueberries	375 mL

For easy slicing, bake a day ahead of serving. Cornbread can be covered and refrigerated for up to 2 days. For longer storage, wrap in freezer wrap and freeze for up to 2 months.

1. Preheat oven to 350°F (180°C). Line 9- x 5-inch (2 L) loaf pan with waxed paper.

2. In mixing bowl, stir together flour, cornmeal, sugar, lemon and orange rind, baking soda and salt.

3. In measuring cup, whisk together eggs, orange juice and oil; stir into dry ingredients just until moistened. Fold in blueberries. Spoon into prepared pan.

4. Bake for 1 to 1-1/4 hours or until toothpick inserted in center comes away clean and loaf is firm to touch.

Per serving (1/2 inch/1 cm)

Calories	138.9
Protein	2.6 g
Carbohydrate	24.8 g
Fat	3.4 g
Calcium	6.7 mg
Dietary Fiber	1.1 g

Percent of calories from:

Carbohydrate:	71%
Protein:	7%
Fat:	22%

Banana Citrus Loaf

Makes an 8½ inch (1.5 L) loaf

When you buy a bunch of bananas, there are always a few that become too ripe for eating. Save them for this recipe. Banana purée replaces milk in this recipe. Serve it sliced on its own or with Pear Butter (page 164) or Tofu Cream Cheese (page 168).

If you don't feel like baking while bananas are at their peak of ripeness, freeze them for future use, skin and all. Simply peel and mash while still partially frozen.

2 cups	cake-and-pastry flour	500 mL
2 tsp	baking powder	10 mL
1 tsp	baking soda	5 mL
½ tsp	each salt and nutmeg	2 mL
1 cup	lightly packed brown sugar	250 mL
½ cup	vegetable oil	125 mL
3	ripe bananas, mashed smooth (1½ cups/375 mL)	3
2	eggs	2
1 tbsp	each grated orange and lemon rind	15 mL

1. Preheat oven to 350°F (180°C). Line 8-1/2 x 4-1/2-inch (1.5 L) loaf pan with waxed paper.

2. In mixing bowl, sift together flour, baking powder, baking soda, salt and nutmeg.

3. In food processor or mixing bowl, combine sugar, oil, bananas, eggs and orange and lemon rind until smooth. Pour into dry ingredients, stirring with fork just until moistened.

4. Spoon into prepared pan. Bake for 55 to 60 minutes or until firm to the touch and toothpick inserted in center comes out clean.

Per serving (1/2 inch/1 cm)

Calories	171.8
Protein	2.0 g
Carbohydrate	25.4 g
Fat	7.2 g
Calcium	20.2 mg
Dietary Fiber	0.5 g

Percent of calories from:

Carbohydrate:	58%
Protein:	5%
Fat:	37%

Glazed Lemon Loaf

A teatime favorite, this is excellent sliced and served with a cup of tea or fruit for dessert or brunch. This loaf freezes well.

Makes an 8½ inch (1.5 L) loaf

If you like, decorate the top of the loaf with slivers of orange and lemon rind before baking.

1½ cups	cake-and-pastry flour	375 mL
1	lemon	1
1 cup	granulated sugar	250 mL
1 tsp	baking soda	5 mL
¼ tsp	salt	1 mL
½ cup	lactose-reduced milk or soy milk	125 mL
⅓ cup	vegetable oil	75 mL
2	eggs	2

1. Preheat oven to 350°F (180°C). Line an 8-1/2 x 4-1/2-inch (1.5 L) loaf pan with waxed paper.

2. Grate rind from lemon to make about 1 tbsp (15 mL). Squeeze juice to make about 1/4 cup (50 mL). Set aside.

3. In mixing bowl, sift together flour, 3/4 cup (175 mL) of the granulated sugar, baking soda and salt.

4. In separate bowl, stir together milk, oil, eggs and lemon rind; stir into dry ingredients just until moistened.

5. Pour into prepared pan. Bake for 45 to 50 minutes or until toothpick inserted in center comes out clean. Let stand about 15 minutes.

6. In small bowl, whisk together remaining sugar and lemon juice; pour over loaf while still warm in pan. Cool completely before slicing.

Per serving (1/2 inch/1 cm)

Calories	130.9
Protein	1.8 g
Carbohydrate	20.3 g
Fat	5.1 g
Calcium	17.1 mg
Dietary Fiber	0.3 g

Percent of calories from:

Carbohydrate:	61%
Protein:	5%
Fat:	34%

Orange, Almond and Apricot Teabread

Makes a 9-inch (2 L) loaf

Apricots and almonds make a classic marriage of flavors. This is one of my favorite recipes, perfect with a cup of tea.

½ cup	chopped unblanched almonds	125 mL
1 cup	dried apricots	250 mL
2 cups	all-purpose flour	500 mL
1 cup	granulated sugar	250 mL
1 tsp	each cream of tartar and baking soda	5 mL
½ tsp	salt	2 mL
¾ cup	orange juice	175 mL
2 tbsp	vegetable oil	25 mL
1 tbsp	grated orange rind	15 mL
½ tsp	almond extract	2 mL
1	egg	1

Sharp kitchen scissors make a fast job of cutting dried apricots.

1. Preheat oven to 350°F (180°C). Line 9- x 5-inch (2 L) loaf pan with waxed paper.

2. Toast almonds on baking sheet for 10 to 15 minutes or until fragrant and brown.

3. Meanwhile, pour boiling water over apricots; let stand about 1 minute. Drain and chop.

4. In mixing bowl, stir together flour, sugar, cream of tartar, baking soda, salt and almonds.

5. In separate bowl, stir together apricots, orange juice, oil, orange rind, almond extract and egg; stir into dry ingredients just until moistened.

6. Spoon into prepared pan. Bake for 55 to 60 minutes or until firm to touch and toothpick inserted in center comes away clean.

Per serving (1/2 inch/1 cm)

Calories	147.5
Protein	2.9 g
Carbohydrate	27.9 g
Fat	3.2 g
Calcium	19.6 mg
Dietary Fiber	1.5 g

Percent of calories from:

Carbohydrate:	74%
Protein:	8%
Fat:	19%

Tropical Coffee Cake

This is an excellent recipe for using up the last overripe banana. Make it in winter when citrus fruits are at their peak and you need to be transported to a southern clime.

Makes 1 bundt cake,
20 servings

1 cup	each whole wheat flour and all-purpose flour	250 mL
¾ cup	granulated sugar	175 mL
1 tsp	each baking soda and baking powder	5 mL
½ tsp	salt	2 mL
1	ripe banana, mashed	1
1 cup	undrained crushed pineapple	250 mL
2	eggs	2
¼ cup	vegetable oil	50 mL
1 tbsp	grated orange rind	15 mL

1. Preheat oven to 350°F (180°C). Grease 10-inch (3 L) bundt pan or spray with nonstick baking spray.

2. In mixing bowl, stir together whole wheat flour, all-purpose flour, granulated sugar, baking soda, baking powder and salt.

3. In separate bowl, beat together banana, pineapple, eggs, oil and orange rind. Add to dry ingredients all at once, stirring just until moistened.

4. Spoon into prepared pan. Bake 50 to 60 minutes or until firm to touch and toothpick inserted in center comes away clean.

Per serving	(1/20th)
Calories	113.1
Protein	2.2 g
Carbohydrate	20.1 g
Fat	3.0 g
Calcium	10.1 mg
Dietary Fiber	1.2 g

Percent of calories from:

Carbohydrate:	69%
Protein:	8%
Fat:	23%

Pear Ginger Cake

Makes 1 bundt cake,
20 servings

Be sure to slice the pears thinly for this recipe. You will find the batter stiff and heavy but the pears give moisture during baking.

1 cup	each whole wheat flour and all-purpose flour	250 mL
1 cup	granulated sugar	250 mL
1 tsp	each baking soda and ginger	5 mL
½ tsp	each nutmeg and salt	2 mL
2 cups	thinly sliced peeled pears	500 mL
½ cup	vegetable oil	125 mL
¼ cup	each toasted chopped almonds and chopped crystallized ginger	50 mL
2	eggs	2
1 tbsp	each grated lemon rind and lemon juice	15 mL

1. Preheat oven to 350°F (180°C). Grease 10-inch (3 L) bundt pan or spray with nonstick baking spray.

2. In mixing bowl, stir together whole wheat flour, all-purpose flour, sugar, baking soda, ground ginger, nutmeg, and salt. Add pears.

3. In small bowl, whisk together oil, almonds, crystallized ginger, eggs, lemon rind and juice; add to dry ingredients all at once, stirring just until moistened.

4. Spoon into prepared pan. Bake for 60 to 70 minutes or until toothpick inserted in center comes away clean. Let stand at least 15 minutes before removing from pan. Cool completely before slicing.

Per serving (1/20th)

Calories	165.2
Protein	2.6 g
Carbohydrate	23.8 g
Fat	7.3 g
Calcium	14.6 mg
Dietary Fiber	2.0 g
	(a source)

Percent of calories from:

Carbohydrate:	56%
Protein:	6%
Fat:	38%

Orange Almond Scone

A scone, traditionally made with cream and butter, is a rich cousin to the tea biscuit. However, this relative boasts orange juice and shortening to produce melt-in-the-mouth perfection. It has the added advantage that you can assemble it up to 12 hours before baking.

2 cups	all-purpose flour	500 mL
½ cup	granulated sugar	125 mL
1 tbsp	grated orange rind	15 mL
2 tsp	baking powder	10 mL
½ tsp	each baking soda and salt	2 mL
⅓ cup	shortening	75 mL
½ cup	orange juice	125 mL
2	eggs	2
¼ cup	chopped almonds	50 mL

1. Preheat oven to 400°F (200°C). Line bottom of 9-inch (1.5 L) round cake pan with waxed paper.

2. In large bowl, stir together flour, all but 1 tbsp (15 mL) of the sugar, orange rind, baking powder, baking soda and salt. With pastry blender or two knives, cut in shortening until in coarse crumbs.

3. In measuring cup, whisk together orange juice and eggs. Reserving 1 tbsp (15 mL) of the orange juice mixture, add remainder to dry ingredients, stirring with fork just until moistened.

4. Spread into prepared pan. Brush with reserved orange juice mixture. Sprinkle evenly with reserved sugar and almonds.

5. Bake for 25 to 30 minutes or until golden brown and firm to touch. Let stand in pan for a few minutes before removing. Run knife around sides of pan to loosen. Cut into wedges and serve warm.

Makes 8 to 12 wedges

If making ahead, cover unbaked scone with plastic wrap. Refrigerate up to 12 hours. Remove from refrigerator 30 minutes before baking.

Per serving	(1/8th)
Calories	283.2
Protein	5.8 g
Carbohydrate	39.2 g
Fat	11.6 g
Calcium	35.7 mg
Dietary Fiber	1.4 g

Percent of calories from:

Carbohydrate:	55%
Protein:	8%
Fat:	37%

Lemon Sesame Twists

Makes 12 biscuits or
1 cake

Shortening does not need to
be refrigerated and is easier
to work with at room
temperature.

Check egg cartons for date
code to use before expiry
date. Discard any eggs
with cracks.

This is a welcome addition to a breadbasket for breakfast, lunch or dinner.

2½ cups	all-purpose flour	625 mL
1 tbsp	each granulated sugar and grated lemon rind	15 mL
2 tsp	baking powder	10 mL
½ tsp	each salt and baking soda	2 mL
½ cup	shortening	125 mL
1 cup	plain yogurt (if tolerated), soy milk or lactose-reduced milk	250 mL
1	egg, beaten	1
	Sesame seeds	

1. Preheat oven to 425°F (220°C). Grease baking sheet or line 9-inch (1.5 L) round cake pan with waxed paper.

2. In mixing bowl, stir together flour, sugar, lemon rind, baking powder, salt and baking soda. Using pastry blender or two knives, cut in shortening until in coarse crumbs.

3. In small bowl, whisk together yogurt and egg. Reserving about 1 tbsp (15 mL) mixture, add remainder into dry ingredients, stirring with fork just until moistened.

4. Divide into 12 equal pieces; roll each into rope and tie into knot, tucking ends under. Place on prepared baking sheet. Or spoon into prepared pan.

5. Brush with reserved egg mixture; sprinkle with sesame seeds.

6. Bake twists for 20 to 25 minutes, cake for 25 to 30 minutes, or until golden brown and firm to touch. May be made a day ahead, or cooled, wrapped well and frozen for up to 3 months. Serve hot or at room temperature.

Per serving (1/12th)

Calories	203.1
Protein	4.5 g
Carbohydrate	23.3 g
Fat	10.0 g
Calcium	65.0 mg
	(a source)
Dietary Fiber	1.2 g

Percent of calories from:

Carbohydrate:	46%
Protein:	9%
Fat:	45%

Sesame Tea Biscuits

After years of experimenting with biscuits, I think this makes the ultimate tender, flaky one, the perfect companion to soups and salads.

2 cups	all-purpose flour	500 mL
2 tsp	each cream of tartar and granulated sugar	10 mL
1 tsp	baking soda	5 mL
½ tsp	salt	2 mL
½ cup	shortening, cubed	125 mL
½ cup	each water and plain yogurt (if tolerated) or 1 cup (250 mL) soy milk or lactose-reduced milk	125 mL
	Sesame seeds	

1. Preheat oven to 425°F (220°C). Grease baking sheet or line with parchment paper.

2. In mixing bowl or food processor, combine flour, cream of tartar, sugar, baking soda and salt. Using pastry blender or steel blade, cut in shortening until in coarse crumbs.

3. If using food processor, transfer to mixing bowl. Using fork, stir water and yogurt, or milk, into dry ingredients just until moistened.

4. Turn out onto lightly floured piece of waxed paper; pat into circle about 1 inch (2.5 cm) thick. Using 2-1/2-inch (6 cm) cookie cutter, cut dough into 9 biscuits; arrange on prepared baking sheet. Or transfer whole circle to baking sheet; cut into wedges. Brush lightly with water; sprinkle with sesame seeds.

5. Bake for about 15 minutes or until golden brown on bottom. Serve immediately or within 1 day. For longer storage, wrap well and freeze in airtight containers for up to 3 months.

Makes 9 large or 12 medium biscuits

Handle dough as little as possible for tender biscuits. To keep dough from sticking to hands and cutter, lightly flour and wipe excess dough from hands and cutter between shaping.

Savory Sesame Biscuits: Add 1/4 cup (50 mL) chopped sun-dried tomatoes and 1 tsp (5 mL) dried basil to flour mixture for a zesty version.

Per serving (1/9th)

Calories	230.7
Protein	4.1 g
Carbohydrate	23.9 g
Fat	13.1 g
Calcium	59.2 mg (a source)
Dietary Fiber	1.5 g

Percent of calories from:

Carbohydrate:	42%
Protein:	7%
Fat:	51%

*C*urrant Scones

Makes 12 to 14 small scones

For super easy biscuits, spoon dough into 10 greased muffin cups and bake for 15 to 20 minutes or until firm to touch. No fuss, no muss!

The dessert version of tea biscuits, scones are usually made with butter, cream or sour cream. This lactose-free version is best served with Quick Strawberry Sauce (page 208) or split and filled with sliced fresh berries as shortcake served with drained Yogurt Sauce (page 167).

2 cups	cake-and-pastry flour	500 mL
2 tbsp	granulated sugar	25 mL
2 tsp	cream of tartar	10 mL
1 tsp	baking soda	5 mL
½ tsp	salt	2 mL
½ cup	shortening, cubed	125 mL
½ cup	each water and plain yogurt (if tolerated) or ⅔ cup (150 mL) lactose-reduced milk	125 mL
½ cup	currants, washed Granulated sugar	125 mL

1. Preheat oven to 425°F (220°C). Grease baking sheet.

2. In mixing bowl or food processor, combine flour, sugar, cream of tartar, baking soda and salt. Using pastry blender or steel blade, cut in shortening until in coarse crumbs.

3. If using food processor, transfer to mixing bowl. Using fork, stir water and yogurt, or lactose-reduced milk, and currants into dry ingredients just until moistened.

4. Turn out onto lightly floured sheet of waxed paper; pat into circle about 1 inch (2.5 cm) thick. Using 1-1/2 inch (4 cm) cookie cutter, cut dough into 12 biscuits; transfer to baking sheet. Or transfer whole circle to baking sheet; cut into wedges. Brush lightly with water; sprinkle with sugar.

5. Bake for 12 to 15 minutes or until golden brown on bottom. Serve immediately or within 1 day. For longer storage, freeze in airtight container for up to 3 months.

Per serving (1/12th)

Calories	160.4
Protein	2.1 g
Carbohydrate	18.4 g
Fat	8.6 g
Calcium	22.1 mg
Dietary Fiber	0.6 g

Percent of calories from:

Carbohydrate:	46%
Protein:	5%
Fat:	49%

Cranberry Apple Muffins

This not-too-sweet muffin is ideal to pack in lunches or munch for breakfast. Fresh or frozen cranberries can be used in this recipe.

Makes 12 large muffins

2 cups	all-purpose flour	500 mL
1 cup	granulated sugar	250 mL
1 tbsp	grated orange rind	15 mL
1 tsp	each cinnamon and baking soda	5 mL
½ tsp	salt	2 mL
¼ tsp	each nutmeg and cardamom	1 mL
1 cup	each unsweetened applesauce and cranberries	250 mL
½ cup	vegetable oil	125 mL
2	eggs	2

Cardamom is a member of the ginger family and has a delightful flavor and fragrance. It is frequently used in Scandinavian baking and East Indian dishes.

1. Preheat oven to 400°F (200°C). Grease or line muffin tins with paper baking cups.

2. In mixing bowl, stir together flour, sugar, orange rind, cinnamon, baking soda, salt, nutmeg and cardamom.

3. In separate bowl, whisk together applesauce, cranberries, oil and eggs; add to dry ingredients all at once, stirring just until moistened.

4. Spoon batter into prepared muffin tins. Bake for 15 to 20 minutes or until muffins spring back when lightly touched.

Per serving

Calories	246.8
Protein	3.3 g
Carbohydrate	36.3 g
Fat	10.2 g
Calcium	12.4 mg
Dietary Fiber	1.4 g

Percent of calories from:

Carbohydrate:	58%
Protein:	5%
Fat:	37%

Good Morning Bran Muffins

Makes 12 large muffins

Here's a hearty muffin to get the morning off to a good start.

1 cup	each whole wheat flour and all-purpose flour	250 mL
1 cup	natural bran	250 mL
1 cup	packed brown sugar	250 mL
1 tsp	each baking powder, baking soda and cinnamon	5 mL
½ tsp	salt	2 mL
1 cup	boiling coffee	250 mL
8 oz	dates, chopped (1¼ cups/300 mL)	250 g
½ cup	molasses	125 mL
¼ cup	vegetable oil	50 mL
1 tbsp	grated orange rind	15 mL
2	eggs, beaten	2

1. Preheat oven to 375°F (190°C). Grease or line muffin tins with paper baking cups.

2. In mixing bowl, stir together whole wheat flour, all-purpose flour, natural bran, sugar, baking powder, baking soda, cinnamon and salt.

3. In separate bowl, pour boiling coffee over dates; stir in molasses, oil and orange rind. Add to dry ingredients all at once. Add eggs; stir just until dry ingredients are moistened.

4. Spoon batter into prepared muffin tins. Bake for 20 to 25 minutes or until firm to touch.

Per serving

Calories	272.8
Protein	4.7 g
Carbohydrate	54.5 g
Fat	6.0 g
Calcium	131.9 mg
	(a source)
Dietary Fiber	3.9 g
	(a high source)

Percent of calories from:

Carbohydrate:	75%
Protein:	6%
Fat:	18%

Double Pumpkin Muffins

Served with Pumpkin Butter recipe (page 164) or spread with honey, these muffins are wonderful packed in a lunch or breakfast to go.

Makes 12 large muffins

1 cup	each all-purpose flour and whole wheat flour	250 mL
1 tsp	each baking soda, baking powder and cinnamon	5 mL
½ tsp	each nutmeg, ground cloves and salt	2 mL
1 cup	pumpkin purée	250 mL
¾ cup	soy milk or lactose-reduced milk	175 mL
½ cup	packed brown sugar	125 mL
½ cup	each pumpkin seeds and washed currants	125 mL
¼ cup	vegetable oil	50 mL
1	egg	1
¼ cup	sesame seeds	50 mL

1. Preheat oven to 375°F (190°C). Grease or line muffin tins with paper baking cups.

2. In mixing bowl, stir together all-purpose flour, whole wheat flour, baking soda, baking powder, cinnamon, nutmeg, cloves and salt.

3. In separate bowl, stir together pumpkin purée, soy milk, sugar, pumpkin seeds, currants, oil, egg and all but 1 tbsp (15 mL) sesame seeds. Add to dry ingredients all at once, stirring just until moistened.

4. Spoon batter into prepared muffin tins. Sprinkle with remaining sesame seeds. Bake for 20 to 25 minutes or until firm to touch and toothpick inserted in center comes out clean.

Per serving

Calories	203.8
Protein	5.6 g
Carbohydrate	27.1 g
Fat	9.0 g
Calcium	58.9 mg
	(a source)
Dietary Fiber	3.6 g
	(a source)

Percent of calories from:

Carbohydrate:	51%
Protein:	11%
Fat:	38%

Banana Bran Muffins with Cinnamon Sugar Topping

Makes 12 large muffins

Serve one of these muffins with a Fruit Smoothie (page 68) for a mini-meal on the run.

1 cup	natural bran	250 mL
1 cup	all-purpose flour	250 mL
½ cup	whole wheat flour	125 mL
1 tsp	each baking soda and baking powder	5 mL
½ tsp	each salt and nutmeg	2 mL
3	large ripe bananas, mashed (1½ cups/375 mL)	3
½ cup	packed brown sugar	125 mL
⅓ cup	vegetable oil	75 mL
2	eggs	2
1 tsp	vanilla	5 mL

Cinnamon Sugar Topping

2 tbsp	brown sugar	25 mL
1 tsp	cinnamon	5 mL

1. Preheat oven to 375°F (190°C). Grease or line muffin tins with paper baking cups.

2. In mixing bowl, stir together bran, all-purpose flour, whole wheat flour, baking soda, baking powder, salt and nutmeg.

3. In separate bowl, combine bananas, sugar, oil, eggs and vanilla; add to dry ingredients all at once, stirring just until moistened. Spoon into prepared muffin tins.

4. Cinnamon Sugar Topping: Combine sugar and cinnamon; sprinkle over batter. Bake for 20 to 25 minutes or until tops spring back when lightly touched.

Per serving

Calories	195.6
Protein	3.9 g
Carbohydrate	31.2 g
Fat	7.4 g
Calcium	26.7 mg
Dietary Fiber	2.1 g
	(a source)

Percent of calories from:

Carbohydrate:	60%
Protein:	8%
Fat:	32%

Carrot, Apple and Almond Muffins

The ever-popular carrot muffin takes on a new guise in this lactose-free version. Applesauce keeps these muffins moist with a minimum of fat and adds a delicate flavor. Serve for breakfast, lunch or nourishing coffee break.

Makes 12 large muffins

For an appealing look, sprinkle a little grated carrot over batter before baking.

1 cup	each whole wheat flour and all-purpose flour	250 mL
1 cup	loosely packed brown sugar	250 mL
2 tsp	cinnamon	10 mL
1 tsp	each baking soda and baking powder	5 mL
½ tsp	salt and nutmeg	2 mL
1 cup	unsweetened applesauce	250 mL
2	large carrots, peeled and coarsely grated (2¼ cups/550 mL)	2
½ cup	toasted chopped almonds	125 mL
¼ cup	vegetable oil	50 mL
2	eggs	2

1. Preheat oven to 375°F (190°C). Grease or line muffin tins with paper baking cups.

2. In mixing bowl, stir together whole wheat flour, all-purpose flour, brown sugar, cinnamon, baking soda, baking powder, salt and nutmeg.

3. In separate bowl, stir together applesauce, carrots, almonds, oil, and eggs. Add to dry ingredients all at once, stirring just until moistened.

4. Spoon batter into prepared muffin tins. Bake for 20 to 25 minutes or until tops spring back when lightly touched. Muffins can be refrigerated for up to 1 week or wrapped well and frozen for up to 3 months.

Per serving

Calories	226.4
Protein	5.1 g
Carbohydrate	37.4 g
Fat	7.2 g
Calcium	58.0 mg
	(a source)
Dietary Fiber	3.6 g
	(a source)

Percent of calories from:

Carbohydrate:	64%
Protein:	9%
Fat:	28%

Yeast Breads

COMMERCIALLY PRODUCED yeast breads may contain milk solids, especially if they are made from a rich dough. Some people with lactose intolerance will be able to cope with bread containing milk products while others will have symptoms. Only you can judge your individual sensitivity. Be sure to check the ingredient listing on the package for milk, milk solids, cheese flavor, whey, curds and some nondairy margarine. Avoid breads containing these products if you are sensitive. Generally, breads that are safe for lactose-intolerant people are Italian or French stick, whole wheat and rye bread.

When making your own breads, you must use a hard wheat flour such as all-purpose or whole wheat, because of its gluten content. Gluten is a protein which gives the bread strength and the ability to rise and stretch. The other essential ingredient is yeast. You can buy it fresh or packaged in dried form. Dry yeast is probably the easiest to work with and is best stored in the refrigerator until the best-before date. You can always tell if yeast is still active by adding the lukewarm water and sugar in the recipe. It will become foamy and have a distinctive beery smell. If it does not do anything, start again with a new yeast. Yeast breads are probably the easiest baking you could ever do. There is no need to feel intimidated— the breads are practically foolproof!

Basic Yeast Bread

This is an easy, versatile recipe using all white or a mixture of whole grain all-purpose flours. It has the flavor and texture of the rich sweet-dough recipes but has no milk or butter added. Because it freezes well for up to six months, make the full recipe using the variations to sample at different times. It makes the best hamburger buns!

3 cups	lukewarm water	750 mL
1 tsp	granulated sugar	5 mL
2	pkg (each 8 g) active dry yeast (traditional) or 2 tbsp (25 mL)	2
½ cup	vegetable oil	125 mL
½ cup	granulated sugar	125 mL
1 tbsp	salt	15 mL
9 cups	all-purpose flour	2.25 L

1. Rinse large mixing bowl with hot tap water; drain. Pour in 1 cup (250 mL) of the lukewarm water; sprinkle with 1 tsp (5 mL) sugar and yeast. Let stand 10 minutes or until foamy and smelling of beer.

2. Whisk in remaining lukewarm water, oil, 1/2 cup (125 mL) sugar and salt. Whisk in about half of the flour, 1 cup (250 mL) at a time. Using wooden spoon or kneading with floured hands, mix in enough of the remaining flour to make stiff dough.

3. Knead dough about 4 minutes or until smooth, satiny, elastic and dough bounces back after finger is pressed into it.

4. Clean bowl and wipe with vegetable oil. Return dough to oiled bowl, turning to grease all over. Allow to rise in warm place, such as turned-off oven with light on, until about doubled in size, 1 to 1-1/2 hours.

5. Punch dough down and shape into any of the following recipes.

Makes 3 loaves or about 4 dozen rolls

The rising procedure may be speeded up by placing bowl in a pan of warm water. Cover bowl with plastic wrap to create a cosy environment. Likewise, the process may be slowed down by placing bowl in a cool spot.

Whole Wheat Bread: Use half whole wheat flour and half all-purpose white flour.

Per serving
1 slice (24 slices/loaf)

Calories	76.3
Protein	1.7 g
Carbohydrate	13.4 g
Fat	1.7 g
Calcium	3.3 mg
Dietary Fiber	0.5 g

Percent of calories from:

Carbohydrate:	71%
Protein:	9%
Fat:	20%

Makes 1 loaf

Braided Loaf

A braided loaf makes an excellent hostess gift.

1. Brush baking sheet with vegetable oil or spray with nonstick baking spray.

2. Using about one-third of the Basic Yeast Bread dough, roll out into 15- x 6-inch (38 x 15 cm) rectangle. Using knife, cut lengthwise into 3 equal strands. Braid and tuck ends under.

3. Using fork, beat 1 egg with spoonful of water; brush over dough. Sprinkle generously with sesame seeds.

4. Place on prepared baking sheet. Let stand in warm place until doubled in size, about 1 hour. Meanwhile, preheat oven to 400°F (200°C).

5. Bake for 20 to 25 minutes or until golden brown and loaf sounds hollow when topped on bottom. Let cool on rack. Keeps well for 2 days or wrap well and freeze for up to 6 months.

Makes 12 pan buns or 18 dinner rolls

Pan Buns

When split and spread with your favorite sandwich filling, pan buns make a tasty change from the usual lunchtime sandwich. If made smaller, they are perfect for dinner rolls.

1. Brush muffin pans with vegetable oil.

2. Using one-third of the Basic Yeast Bread dough, divide into 12 equal portions for lunchtime buns or 18 for dinner rolls. Roll each into ball. Dip into bowl of sesame seeds.

3. Place each ball, sesame seed side up, in muffin pan. Let stand in warm place until doubled in size, about 1 hour. Meanwhile, preheat oven to 400°F (200°C).

4. Bake for 12 to 15 minutes or until golden brown and buns sound hollow when tapped on bottom.

Bow Knots

1. Brush baking sheet with vegetable oil or spray with nonstick baking spray.

2. Using one-third of the Basic Yeast Bread dough, divide into 12 equal portions. Shape each into 6-inch (15 mL) long rope. Tie loosely into knot and tuck ends under. Dip into bowl of sesame seeds.

3. Place each knot about 2 inches (10 cm) apart on prepared baking sheet. Let stand in warm place until doubled in size, 45 to 60 minutes. Meanwhile, preheat oven to 400°F (200°C).

4. Bake for 12 to 15 minutes or until golden brown and bow knots sound hollow when tapped on bottom.

Hamburger Buns

These moist, slightly sweet buns contribute to a superb hamburger experience.

1. Brush baking sheet with vegetable oil or spray with nonstick baking spray. Using one-third of the Basic Yeast Bread dough, divide into 8 equal portions. Shape each into ball.

2. Using fork, beat 1 egg with spoonful of water; brush over dough. Dip into bowl of sesame seeds.

3. Place each bun about 1 inch (2.5 cm) apart on prepared baking sheet. Let stand in warm place until doubled in size, about 1 hour. Meanwhile, preheat oven to 400°F (200°C).

4. Bake for 12 to 15 minutes or until golden brown and buns sound hollow when tapped on bottom.

Makes 8 croissants

Croissant Shaped Rolls

1. Brush baking sheet with vegetable oil or spray with nonstick baking spray.

2. Using one-third of the Basic Yeast Bread dough and with rolling pin, roll out into circle about 1/4 inch (5 mm) thick. Using knife, cut into 8 wedges. Starting from outside edge, roll dough into center; curve ends inwards.

3. Using fork, beat 1 egg with spoonful of water; brush over dough.

4. Place on prepared baking sheet. Let stand in warm place until doubled in size, about 1 hour. Meanwhile, preheat oven to 400°F (200°C).

5. Bake for 12 to 15 minutes or until golden brown and rolls sound hollow when tapped on bottom.

Egg Wash: Egg wash in a recipe acts as a type of glue, usually to make seeds stick. Egg wash also gives a golden sheen to baked goods. To make egg wash, combine beaten egg with a spoonful of water. Use a pastry brush to paint egg wash onto the baked goods. Egg wash may be kept covered and refrigerated for up to 1 day.

*H*erbed Spiral Loaf

A fragrant loaf spiralled with fresh chopped herbs makes a pretty slice and sight.

Makes a 9-inch (2 L) loaf

Herb Filling

2 tbsp	extra virgin olive oil	25 mL
1 cup	chopped green onions (about 4)	250 mL
1 cup	chopped fresh parsley	250 mL
2 tbsp	each dried basil and tarragon	25 mL
2	cloves garlic, minced	2
1 tbsp	fresh lemon juice	15 mL
One-third	Basic Yeast Bread Dough (page 152)	One-third
	Egg wash (page 155)	
	Sesame seeds	

1. Brush 9-inch (2 L) loaf pan with vegetable oil or spray with nonstick baking spray.

2. In skillet, heat oil over medium heat; cook onions, parsley, basil, tarragon and garlic, covered, until herbs are softened, about 3 minutes. Stir in lemon juice.

3. Using rolling pin, roll out Basic Yeast Bread dough into 15- x 10-inch (38 x 25 cm) rectangle. Spread with herbs to within 1 inch (2.5 cm) of border. Starting from short end, roll up like jelly roll, tucking ends under. Brush with egg wash; sprinkle with sesame seeds.

4. Transfer to prepared loaf pan. Let stand in warm place until doubled in size, about 1 hour.

5. Bake for 25 minutes or until golden brown.

Per serving	(1/16th)
Calories	56.3
Protein	1.2 g
Carbohydrate	7.6 g
Fat	2.5 g
Calcium	20.1 mg
Dietary Fiber	0.8 g

Percent of calories from:

Carbohydrate:	53%
Protein:	8%
Fat:	39%

Swedish Tea Ring

Makes 1 coffee cake,
16 servings

One-third	Basic Yeast Bread dough (page 152)	One-third
	Egg wash (page 155)	
½ cup	packed brown sugar	125 mL
½ cup	chopped toasted almonds	125 mL
½ cup	raisins or washed currants	125 mL
1 tsp	cinnamon	5 mL
½ tsp	nutmeg	2 mL

Glaze

This is always a hit for brunch or with a cup of coffee.

¾ cup	sifted icing sugar	175 mL
2 tbsp	lemon juice	25 mL

1. Brush baking sheet with vegetable oil or spray with nonstick baking spray.

2. Using rolling pin, roll out dough into 15- x 10-inch (38 x 25 cm) rectangle. Using pastry brush, paint dough with egg wash.

3. In small bowl, stir together sugar, almonds, raisins, cinnamon and nutmeg; sprinkle evenly over rectangle to within 1 inch (2.5 cm) of border. Starting from short end, roll up like jelly roll. Form into circle.

4. Place on prepared baking sheet. Using scissors, slash dough at 2-inch (10 cm) intervals three-quarters of the way through ring. Alternately arrange one piece in and one piece out of circle. Cover loosely with tea towel. Let stand in warm place until doubled in size, about 1 hour. Meanwhile, preheat oven to 400°F (200°C).

5. Bake for 25 to 30 minutes or until golden brown and firm to touch. Let cool.

6. Glaze: In small bowl, whisk together icing sugar and lemon juice; drizzle over cooled ring.

Per serving	(1/16th)
Calories	180.9
Protein	3.2 g
Carbohydrate	35.4 g
Fat	3.4 g
Calcium	20.5 mg
Dietary Fiber	1.3 g

Percent of calories from:

Carbohydrate:	77%
Protein:	7%
Fat:	16%

Easy Health Bread

This super-simple loaf requires a minimum of kneading and as a result is a coarse-grained bread that's ideal for toast or sandwiches. Bake two, one to eat now and another to freeze for future use.

Makes two 9-inch (2 L) loaves

3 cups	lukewarm water	750 mL
2 tsp	granulated sugar	10 mL
2	pkg (each 8 g) active dry yeast or 2 tbsp (25 mL)	2
¼ cup	molasses or liquid honey	50 mL
¼ cup	packed brown sugar	50 mL
¼ cup	vegetable oil	50 mL
1 tbsp	salt	15 mL
6 cups	whole wheat flour	1.5 L
1 cup	natural bran	250 mL
½ cup	wheat germ	125 mL
½ cup	quick-cooking rolled oats	125 mL
½ cup	mixed seeds such as sesame, poppy or pumpkin seeds	125 mL

1. Grease two 9- x 5-inch (2 L) loaf pans.

2. Rinse large mixing bowl with hot tap water; drain. Pour in lukewarm water; sprinkle with sugar and yeast. Let stand 10 minutes or until foamy and smelling of beer.

3. Whisk in molasses, brown sugar, oil and salt. Whisk in 3 cups (750 mL) of the flour, bran, wheat germ, rolled oats and seeds. Beat in enough of the remaining flour to make heavy, slightly wet dough. Flour hands and knead 1 to 2 minutes.

4. Place dough in greased bowl, turning to grease all over. Cover with tea towel or plastic wrap. Let stand in warm spot until doubled in size, about 1 hour.

5. Punch down dough. Knead about 1 minute. Divide in half; shape into loaves and place in prepared pans. Cover loosely with tea towel; let rise in warm spot until doubled in size, about 45 minutes. Meanwhile, preheat oven to 375°F (190°C).

6. Bake for 45 to 55 minutes or until deep golden brown and loaf sounds hollow when tapped on bottom. Let cool on rack about 20 minutes before removing from pans to racks.

Per serving
(1 slice/24 per loaf)

Calories	92.4
Protein	3.5 g
Carbohydrate	15.4 g
Fat	2.7 g
Calcium	32.6 mg
Dietary Fiber	2.7 g
	(a source)

Percent of calories from:

Carbohydrate:	62%
Protein:	14%
Fat:	24%

Celebration Bread

Wonderfully rich without the usual butter and milk, this sticky dough produces a moist tender bread. It can be shaped into hot cross buns for Easter, into a German stollen or easily spooned into a bundt pan for a special Christmas coffee cake. Once baked and well wrapped, it keeps frozen for up to six months.

1½ cups	lukewarm water	375 mL
1	pkg (8 g) active dry yeast (traditional) or 1 tbsp (15 mL)	1
1 tsp	granulated sugar	5 mL
½ cup	granulated sugar	125 mL
½ cup	vegetable oil	125 mL
1	egg	1
1 cup	raisins	250 mL
½ cup	currants, washed, or candied peel	125 mL
½ cup	toasted chopped almonds	125 mL
1 tbsp	grated lemon rind	15 mL
2 tsp	salt	10 mL
1½ tsp	cinnamon	7 mL
½ tsp	each cloves, cardamom and nutmeg	2 mL
4 cups	all-purpose flour	1 L
	Egg wash (page 155)	

Glaze

¾ cup	sifted icing sugar	175 mL
2 tbsp	fresh lemon juice	25 mL
	Almonds (optional)	

Makes 1 loaf

If a 14-cup (3.5 L) bundt pan is unavailable, use a regular 12-cup (3 L) bundt and one (8-1/2- x 4-1/2-inch/1.5 L) loaf pan instead.

1. Rinse large mixing bowl with hot tap water; drain. Pour in 1/2 cup (125 mL) of the lukewarm water; sprinkle with yeast and 1 tsp (5 mL) sugar. Let stand 10 minutes or until foamy and smelling of beer.

2. Gradually whisk in remaining water, sugar, oil, egg, raisins, currants, almonds, lemon rind, salt, cinnamon, cloves, cardamom and nutmeg. Whisk in flour, 1 cup (250 mL) at a time, using wooden spoon when dough becomes heavy. Beat vigorously with spoon or knead with well-floured hands until well combined. Dough should be moist.

3. Place in greased bowl, turning to grease all over. Cover loosely with tea towel. Let stand in warm spot until doubled in size, 1-1/2 to 2 hours.

4. Grease baking sheet or 14-cup (3.5 L) bundt pan.

5. Punch dough down. Knead with floured hands for 1 to 2 minutes. For stollen, form into oval and fold over lengthwise. For hot cross buns, divide into 16 portions and shape into balls. Place on prepared baking sheet. For bundt, place in prepared bundt.

6. Let rise in warm spot until doubled in size, 1 to 1-1/2 hours. Meanwhile, preheat oven to 375°F (190°C). Brush dough with egg wash.

7. Bake for 30 to 35 minutes for stollen, 20 to 25 minutes for buns, 45 to 50 minutes for bundt or until golden brown and bread sounds hollow when tapped on bottom. Cool on racks.

8. Glaze: In small bowl, whisk together icing sugar and lemon juice; drizzle over cooled bread. For hot cross buns, drizzle to make cross. For stollen or bundt, decorate with almonds if desired.

To speed rising action of dough, place bowl with the dough in a larger bowl of warm water. Cover with plastic wrap. Dough should be doubled in size in double-quick time!

Per serving
(1 slice/24 per loaf)

Calories	192.9
Protein	3.4 g
Carbohydrate	32.3 g
Fat	6.1 g
Calcium	23.2 mg
Dietary Fiber	1.5 g

Percent of calories from:

Carbohydrate:	65%
Protein:	7%
Fat:	28%

Sauces and Spreads

MILK, CREAM, cheese or butter are the usual ingredients for these basic recipes. Some or all of these may cause problems to lactose-intolerant people. These lactose-free versions feature alternative ingredients with delectable results.

Pumpkin Butter

This is wonderful spread for pumpkin muffins or seed and nut bread.

2 cups	pumpkin purée	500 mL
½ cup	apple juice	125 mL
¼ cup	molasses	50 mL
1 tbsp	packed brown sugar	15 mL
½ tsp	cinnamon	2 mL
¼ tsp	each ground cloves and ginger	1 mL
Pinch	salt	Pinch

1. In large stainless steel saucepan, combine pumpkin purée, apple juice, molasses, brown sugar, cinnamon, cloves, ginger and salt.

2. Bring to boil; reduce heat and simmer, uncovered, about 5 minutes or until thickened. Cool. Spoon into jar, cover and refrigerate up to 5 days.

Makes about 2 cups (500 mL)

Per serving (2 tbsp/25 mL)

Calories	28.0
Protein	0.3 g
Carbohydrate	7.0 g
Fat	0.1 g
Calcium	44.4 mg
Dietary Fiber	0.6 g

Percent of calories from:

Carbohydrate:	92%
Protein:	5%
Fat:	3%

Pear Butter

Pear butter is a delectable, thick, spiced spread for pancakes, toast and muffins or a condiment with pork or poultry. It's so yummy, you just might eat it by the spoonful too!

4	pears, peeled, cored and diced	4
1 cup	water	250 mL
½ cup	liquid honey	125 mL
2 tbsp	fresh lemon juice	25 mL
1	strip lemon peel	1
1	cinnamon stick	1

Makes about 2 cups (500 mL)

Per serving (2 tbsp/25 mL)

Calories	42.5
Protein	0.1 g
Carbohydrate	11.4 g
Fat	0.0 g
Calcium	3.3 mg
Dietary Fiber	0.4 g

Percent of calories from:

Carbohydrate:	99%
Protein:	1%
Fat:	0%

When a recipe specifies stainless steel saucepans, it's because the metal will not react with the acid of the ingredients. A glass saucepan would work just as well.

1. In stainless steel saucepan, combine pears, water, honey, lemon juice, lemon peel and cinnamon stick. Bring to boil; simmer, stirring, over medium heat about 15 minutes or until pears are very tender.

2. Discard peel and cinnamon stick. Purée in food processor or beat with fork until smooth.

3. Spoon into jar, cover and refrigerate for up to 1 week or freeze for up to 3 months.

Makes about 2 cups
(500 mL)

Apple Butter

An old-fashioned recipe, this spicy spread is the perfect companion to pancakes or pork.

You won't need butter when you have these flavorful spreads. Be sure to make pear butter in the autumn when pears are cheap and plentiful. Each pear variety will give a different flavor and texture to the spread.

4 cups	apples, peeled, cored and chopped (about 6 medium)	1 L
2 cups	apple juice	500 mL
⅓ cup	liquid honey	75 mL
½ tsp	cinnamon	2 mL
¼ tsp	ground cloves	1 mL

1. In stainless steel saucepan, combine apples, apple juice, honey, cinnamon and cloves.

2. Bring to boil; reduce heat and simmer, uncovered, 20 to 25 minutes or until soft and mushy. For a super smooth texture, purée in blender or beat with fork. Serve hot or cold. Keeps refrigerated in airtight container for up to 1 week.

Per serving (2 tbsp/25 mL)

Calories	56.7
Protein	0.2 g
Carbohydrate	14.7 g
Fat	0.2 g
Calcium	5.7 mg
Dietary Fiber	0.4 g

Percent of calories from:
Carbohydrate:	96%
Protein:	1%
Fat:	3%

Lemon Butter

This classic, rich, creamy and intensely flavored spread is ideal for tea breads, jelly roll slices as a filling for tarts and meringues.

Makes about 1 cup
(250 mL)

1 cup	granulated sugar	250 mL
½ cup	fresh lemon juice	125 mL
1 tbsp	grated lemon rind	15 mL
2	eggs	2

1. In mixing bowl, whisk together sugar, lemon juice, lemon rind and eggs until smooth.

2. Pour into stainless steel saucepan; cook, whisking, over medium heat until just bubbling, thickened and smooth, about 10 minutes. Let cool.

3. Spoon into jar, cover and refrigerate for up to 1 week or freeze for up to 1 month.

Variation:

Lime Butter: Substitute lime juice and lime rind for lemon juice and lemon rind.

Citrus Butter: Use a combination of lemon, lime and orange to make up the amounts of juice and rind in the recipe.

Per serving (1 tbsp/15 mL)

Calories	109.5
Protein	0.7 g
Carbohydrate	26.3 g
Fat	0.7 g
Calcium	6.1 mg
Dietary Fiber	0.0 g

Percent of calories from:

Carbohydrate:	92%
Protein:	2%
Fat:	6%

Yogurt Sauce

Makes 1 cup (250 mL)

No one will ever guess the simplicity and healthy base of this delicious creamy sauce. If time is tight, simply stir the brown sugar and flavoring into the undrained yogurt for an instant sauce. It can be served with fresh berries, over puddings or as a sauce for cakes.

Many people with lactose intolerance find that they can digest yogurt with natural bacteria. The bacteria helps break down the lactose. If you can digest yogurt, try to incorporate it into your diet as a calcium source.

2 cups	plain yogurt	500 mL
¼ cup	packed brown sugar	50 mL
1 tbsp	dark rum, amaretto liqueur or vanilla	15 mL

1. Spoon yogurt into sieve lined with two layers of cheesecloth or into coffee filter over bowl. Cover and refrigerate about 4 hours or overnight or until reduced by about half.

2. In mixing bowl, stir together reduced yogurt, sugar and rum until well combined. Serve immediately or cover and refrigerate for up to 1 day.

Per serving (1 tbsp/15 mL)

Calories	28.5
Protein	1.5 g
Carbohydrate	4.9 g
Fat	0.0 g
Calcium	53.9 mg
Dietary Fiber	0.0 g

Percent of calories from:
Carbohydrate:	69%
Protein:	21%
Fat:	1%

Tofu Cream Cheese

Use this as a spread for bagels, as a dip or sandwich filling.

1	pkg (10.25 oz/290 g) silken firm tofu	1
1 tbsp	each fresh lemon juice and vegetable oil	15 mL
¼ tsp	salt	1 mL

1. Using sieve, drain tofu.

2. Using food processor, purée together drained tofu, lemon juice, oil and salt until smooth.

3. Cover and refrigerate in airtight container for up to 3 days.

Per serving (1 tbsp/15 mL)

Calories	18.7
Protein	1.2 g
Carbohydrate	0.6 g
Fat	1.3 g
Calcium	5.4 mg
Dietary Fiber	0.0 g

Percent of calories from:

Carbohydrate:	12%
Protein:	25%
Fat:	63%

Finales

Simple Pleasures

WARM AND cosy comfort desserts like puddings, pies and crisps served with milk, cream or ice cream are old standbys. By substituting fruit juice for milk and modifying sauces, lactose-intolerant people can still keep them as favorites.

Basic Custard

Custard is one of the original comfort foods. When made with milk, it is considered a calcium-rich dessert that's nutritious for children. But there is nothing to say custard has to be made with milk (although that version is below). Try any variety of juices, even coffee, for a wonderful sauce over fruit, cake or in a trifle.

Makes about 1½ cups
(375 mL) or 4 servings

½ cup	granulated sugar	125 mL
4	egg yolks	4
1 cup	orange juice	250 mL

1. In heavy stainless steel saucepan, whisk together sugar and yolks until smooth. Gradually whisk in orange juice.

2. Cook over medium heat until thickened, about 5 minutes, whisking frequently to prevent curdling.

Variation:

Lactose-Free Custard: For a milk-based custard, use lactose-reduced milk or soy milk to replace orange juice; add 1 tsp (5 mL) vanilla.

Per serving

Calories	181.9
Protein	3.2 g
Carbohydrate	31.6 g
Fat	5.2 g
Calcium	28.5 mg
Dietary Fiber	0.2 g

Percent of calories from:

Carbohydrate:	68%
Protein:	7%
Fat:	25%

Sesame Crunch

Makes about 30 squares

An ideal lunchtime treat, this square packs a powerful calcium punch from sesame seeds and almonds. It's a fun recipe for children to help with, especially when they can mix the ingredients with their hands.

Toast almonds and sesame seeds on a baking dish at 350°F (180°C) 12 to 15 minutes or until golden brown and fragrant.

2 cups	corn flakes	500 mL
1 cup	quick-cooking rolled oats	250 mL
½ cup	each chopped toasted almonds and sesame seeds	125 mL
½ cup	liquid honey	125 mL
½ cup	packed brown sugar	125 mL

1. Preheat oven to 350°F (180°C). Grease 8-inch (2 L) square baking dish or spray with nonstick baking spray.

2. In mixing bowl, crush corn flakes with hands or base of small bowl until in coarse crumbs. Stir in rolled oats, almonds, sesame seeds, honey and sugar until well combined. Pack firmly into prepared dish.

3. Bake for 25 minutes or until golden brown. While still warm, cut into squares with sharp knife. Let cool completely before removing from pan.

Per serving   (1 square)

Calories	72.5
Protein	1.6 g
Carbohydrate	12.1 g
Fat	2.5 g
Calcium	37.4 mg
Dietary Fiber	1.0 g

Percent of calories from:

Carbohydrate:	63%
Protein:	8%
Fat:	29%

Bread Pudding

This dressed-up version of a popular classic has a fanciful meringue topping that makes it special enough to serve to guests as well as family.

¾ cup	raisins	175 mL
6 cups	cubed bread (about 8 slices)	1.5 L
3 cups	lactose-reduced milk or soy milk	750 mL
4	egg yolks	4
½ cup	packed brown sugar	125 mL
1 tsp	each vanilla and cinnamon	5 mL
¼ tsp	each salt and grated nutmeg	1 mL
	Basic Custard (page 172)	

Topping

4	egg whites	4
Pinch	salt	Pinch
¼ cup	granulated sugar	50 mL
1 tsp	vanilla	5 mL
2 tbsp	toasted chopped almonds	25 mL

1. Preheat oven to 350°F (180°C). Grease 12-cup (3 L) baking dish.

2. In small bowl, pour boiling water over raisins.

3. Meanwhile, in mixing bowl, stir together bread, milk, egg yolks, brown sugar, vanilla, cinnamon, salt and nutmeg. Drain raisins; stir into bread mixture.

4. Topping: In another bowl using electric mixer, beat egg whites and salt until soft peaks form. Gradually beat in sugar and vanilla until stiff peaks form.

5. Spoon bread mixture into prepared dish; spread meringue evenly over top, making decorative swirls with knife. Sprinkle with almonds.

6. Bake for 50 to 60 minutes or until meringue is golden brown and bread seems moist but set. Serve with Basic Custard.

Per serving
(Bread Pudding only)

Calories	323.6
Protein	10.1 g
Carbohydrate	56.5 g
Fat	6.9 g
Calcium	173.8 mg
	(a high source)
Dietary Fiber	1.0 g

Percent of calories from:
Carbohydrate:	69%
Protein:	12%
Fat:	19%

Creamy Stove Top Rice Pudding

Makes 6 servings

It's hard to believe that a dessert so good can be nutritious too! In fact, it's so healthy, you could eat it for breakfast.

The creaminess in this rice pudding comes from a combination of short grain rice, fruit juice and egg to give it a custardlike texture and smooth taste.

Italian short grain rice, available in supermarkets, works well in this dessert.

3 cups	water	750 mL
1	cinnamon stick	1
½ cup	short grain rice	125 mL
1 cup	apple juice	250 mL
⅓ cup	loosely packed brown sugar	75 mL
1 tsp	vanilla	5 mL
¼ tsp	grated nutmeg	1 mL
2	eggs, beaten	2
⅓ cup	currants, washed, or raisins	75 mL

1. In saucepan over high heat, bring 2 cups (500 mL) of the water and cinnamon stick to boil. Stir in rice. Return to boil; reduce heat and simmer 35 to 40 minutes until rice is very tender and water has been absorbed.

2. Stir in remaining water, apple juice, sugar, vanilla and nutmeg. Cook, covered, over low heat about 10 minutes or until rice is creamy.

3. Beat in eggs and currants. Cook, stirring, about 2 minutes. Discard cinnamon stick. For best flavor, serve warm.

Per serving

Calories	160.2
Protein	3.1 g
Carbohydrate	32.4 g
Fat	2.1 g
Calcium	32.2 mg
Dietary Fiber	0.7 g

Percent of calories from:

Carbohydrate:	81%
Protein:	8%
Fat:	12%

Caramelized Peach Rice Gâteau

Although this is supposed to serve six, I must admit to polishing off more than my generous share! For lovers of rice pudding, this chic version is certainly worth making for guests. It should be served at room temperature with a garnish of sliced peaches and a sprig of mint.

Makes 6 servings

2 cups	water	500 mL
½ cup	short grain rice	125 mL
1 cup	peach cocktail	250 mL
½ cup	granulated sugar	125 mL
1 tsp	grated lemon rind	5 mL
½ tsp	almond extract	2 mL
¼ tsp	grated nutmeg	1 mL
2	eggs, beaten	2

Short grain rice is used for desserts to give a creamy pudding texture, one that sticks together. Long grain rice tends to be more separate and as such is ideal for rice pilafs.

Topping

2 tbsp	chopped toasted almonds	25 mL
2 tbsp	packed brown sugar	25 mL

1. Preheat oven to 350°F (180°C). Grease 6-cup (1.5 L) shallow baking dish.

2. In saucepan, bring water to boil. Stir in rice. Return to boil; reduce heat, cover and simmer 35 to 40 minutes or until rice is very tender and water has been absorbed.

3. In mixing bowl, whisk together peach cocktail, sugar, lemon rind, almond extract, nutmeg and eggs. Gradually whisk in cooked rice. Pour into prepared baking dish.

Peach cocktail is a peach drink made from a variety of fruit juices and peach purée with a delicate taste that says "peach." It is available in the juice section of grocery stores.

4. Bake, uncovered, 55 to 60 minutes or until set. Mixture will jiggle in center but will firm up on cooling. Let stand for 1 hour. Can be made up to 4 hours before serving.

5. Topping: Sprinkle top evenly with almonds and brown sugar. Broil until sugar has caramelized, about 2 minutes. Serve at once.

Per serving

Calories	191.3
Protein	3.6 g
Carbohydrate	37.1 g
Fat	3.5 g
Calcium	30.0 mg
Dietary Fiber	0.6 g

Percent of calories from:

Carbohydrate:	77%
Protein:	7%
Fat:	16%

Fruit Crisp

Whenever I need a speedy dessert to satisfy friends or family, fruit crisp comes to mind. By choosing different fruits and altering toppings, I can come up with quite a glamorous dessert in minutes. My buttery crisp of the past has been altered to make a crunchy topping with honey to balance the flavors of old. Serve this nutritious treat in small servings.

Makes 4 to 6 servings

6 cups	sliced, peeled fruit	1.5 L
1 cup	granulated sugar	250 mL
1 tbsp	grated lemon or orange rind	15 mL
1 tsp	cinnamon	5 mL

Crisp Topping

1 cup	each all-purpose flour and quick-cooking rolled oats	250 mL
½ cup	each liquid honey and packed brown sugar	125 mL
¼ cup	vegetable oil	50 mL
¼ cup	chopped toasted almonds	50 mL
½ tsp	ground cardamom or cinnamon	2 mL
Pinch	salt	Pinch

Apples, pears and peaches are popular choices for crisps. Cranberries, blueberries, strawberries and raspberries are all delectable additions. One apple will yield about 1 cup (250 mL) peeled, cored and sliced fruit.

1. Preheat oven to 375°F (190°C). Grease 8-cup (2 L) baking dish or spray with nonstick baking spray.

2. In mixing bowl, stir together fruit, sugar, lemon rind and cinnamon. Arrange in prepared dish.

3. Crisp Topping: In same mixing bowl, stir together flour, rolled oats, honey, sugar, oil, nuts, cardamom and salt. Sprinkle evenly over fruit.

4. Bake for 40 to 45 minutes or until fruit is tender and crisp is bubbly.

Per serving (1/6 recipe)

Calories	611.0
Protein	7.0 g
Carbohydrate	123.2 g
Fat	13.4 g
Calcium	65.0 mg
	(a source)
Dietary Fiber	4.3 g
	(a high source)

Percent of calories from:

Carbohydrate:	77%
Protein:	4%
Fat:	19%

Lactose-Free Shortbread

Makes about 4 dozen

Shortbread relies upon the unique flavor of butter for its magnificence. This lactose-free version uses shortening for texture and brown sugar and vanilla for flavor. Taste these to see if they don't measure up to the traditional cookie!

Parchment paper or silicone paper makes removing baked goods from baking pans easy. It is available in many supermarkets and cookery stores.

2 cups	all-purpose flour	500 mL
½ cup	rice flour	125 mL
½ tsp	salt	2 mL
1 cup	shortening	250 mL
⅔ cup	packed brown sugar	150 mL
2 tsp	vanilla	10 mL

1. Preheat oven to 350°F (180°C). Line baking sheet with parchment paper.

2. In mixing bowl, stir together all-purpose flour, rice flour and salt.

3. In separate bowl using electric mixer, beat together shortening, sugar and vanilla until fluffy. Gradually beat in flour mixture, 1/2 cup (125 mL) at a time, scraping down bowl occasionally.

4. Roll dough out between 2 sheets of waxed paper to 1/4-inch (5 mm) thickness. Remove top layer of paper. Using fancy cookie cutter, cut out cookies and arrange on prepared baking sheet. Reroll dough and continue to cut out until all dough is used.

5. Bake 20 to 25 minutes or until golden brown.

Per serving (1 shortbread)

Calories	71.9
Protein	0.6 g
Carbohydrate	7.5 g
Fat	4.3 g
Calcium	3.0 mg
Dietary Fiber	0.2 g

Percent of calories from:

Carbohydrate:	42%
Protein:	4%
Fat:	54%

Basic Sponge

This is one of the easiest, most versatile lactose-free cake recipes that bakers can have in their repertoire. Depending on the shape of pan used, you have a different creation. Every Christmas I use it as a jelly roll for the traditional Yule Log. Each spring it is transformed with the addition of lemon zest, lemon filling and a sprinkling of strawberries to celebrate Easter. It can also be made into a layer cake—filled with raspberry jam and sprinkled with icing sugar for an everyday treat. The variations are endless, as you will discover when you start concocting your own.

Makes one 9-inch (23 cm) round cake or one 15- x 10-inch (2 L) jelly roll

3	eggs	3
1 cup	granulated sugar	250 mL
⅓ cup	water	75 mL
1 tsp	vanilla	5 mL
1 cup	all-purpose flour	250 mL
1 tsp	baking powder	5 mL
¼ tsp	salt	1 mL
	Icing sugar (optional)	

1. For cake: Preheat oven to 350°F (180°C). Line bottom of 9-inch (1.5 L) round cake pan with waxed paper. For jelly roll: Preheat oven to 375°F (190°C). Line bottom of 15- x 10-inch (2 L) jelly roll pan with waxed paper.

2. In mixing bowl using electric mixer, beat eggs until light in color. Gradually beat in sugar until thick and pale colored. Beat in water and vanilla.

3. Sift flour, baking powder and salt over egg mixture; beat until combined. Pour into prepared pan.

4. Bake cake for 25 to 30 minutes, or until golden brown; bake jelly roll for 15 to 20 minutes, or until golden brown.

Per serving　(1/8th recipe)

Basic sponge:
Calories	183.7
Protein	3.5 g
Carbohydrate	37.4 g
Fat	2.3 g
Calcium	19.7 mg
Dietary Fiber	0.5 g

Percent of calories from:
Carbohydrate:	81%
Protein:	8%
Fat:	11%

5. Let stand 10 minutes before inverting onto cooling rack and removing waxed paper. For jelly roll, sift icing sugar over clean tea towel. Invert the jelly roll pan over towel. Remove pan and gently remove waxed paper. Roll up jelly roll along short end in tea towel. Cool completely. Unroll and remove towel to fill.

Variations:

Chocolate Jelly Roll or Sponge Layer Cake: Reduce flour to 3/4 cup (175 mL) and use 1/4 cup (50 mL) unsweetened cocoa powder. Fill with Chocolate Cream Filling (page 207) and spread with Cappuccino Sauce (page 209).

Makes 8 servings

Unroll Chocolate Jelly Roll and spread with Coffee Cream Filling (page 207, variation); reroll. Trim ends at an angle; place cut pieces on top of either end of the "log" as "knots." Spread outside of log with thin layer of Cappuccino Sauce (page 209). Dab remaining coffee filling at the end and on top of knots for "snow." Carefully transfer to serving platter and garnish base with fresh greenery from evergreen.

Apple Jelly Roll or Sponge Layer Cake: Substitute apple juice for water and add 1/2 tsp (2 mL) ground cinnamon. Fill with Apple Butter (page 165) and sift icing sugar over surface. Decorate with apple slices dipped into lemon juice.

Citrus Jelly Roll or Sponge Layer Cake: Substitute orange juice for water and add 1 tbsp (15 mL) each grated lemon and orange rind. Fill with Lemon or Lime Butter (page 166) and use it to pipe lemon rosettes onto surface. Garnish with kiwifruit or strawberries.

Per serving   (1/8th recipe)

Yule Log:

Calories	443.0
Protein	15.8 g
Carbohydrate	80.8 g
Fat	9.4 g
Calcium	70.9 mg
	(a source)
Dietary Fiber	2.7 g
	(a source)

Percent of calories from:

Carbohydrate:	68%
Protein:	13%
Fat:	18%

Basic Meringue

Here's another lactose-free, low-fat recipe that can take many guises. Serve small meringues piled in a glass bowl drizzled with Cappuccino Sauce (page 209) or make the dessert meringues and fill with a spoonful of Lemon Butter (page 166) and top with sliced strawberries. Or make into layers and spread with Lemon Butter; sprinkle with sliced berries and stack for a torte.

4	egg whites	4
½ tsp	cream of tartar	2 mL
1 cup	granulated sugar	250 mL
1 tsp	vanilla	5 mL

1. Preheat oven to 300°F (150°C). Line baking sheet with parchment paper.

2. In mixing bowl using electric mixer, beat egg whites and cream of tartar until stiff peaks form. Gradually beat in sugar, a spoonful at a time, until stiff peaks form. Fold in vanilla.

3. For small meringues, spoon a heaped teaspoon onto baking sheet, forming into peak and leaving 2 inches (5 cm) space between each. For dessert meringues, spoon about 1/4 cup (50 mL) onto baking sheet; using back of dampened spoon, indent center. For torte, use 9-inch (23 cm) plate as template and draw 3 circles on parchment. Spread even quantities of meringue onto circles, leaving 1-inch (2.5 cm) border uncovered.

4. Bake small meringues or tortes 25 to 30 minutes, large meringues 30 to 35 minutes, or until golden brown. Turn oven off and let cool completely in oven. May be made up to one week in advance and stored in dry place such as cake tin. Do not store in plastic or meringue will become soft. May be frozen for longer storage.

Makes 24 small or
8 dessert meringues,
or 3 torte layers

Lining baking sheets with parchment paper, available in some supermarkets and kitchen stores, makes removal of meringue a breeze.

Per serving (1/24th)

Calories	35.0
Protein	0.5 g
Carbohydrate	8.4 g
Fat	0.0 g
Calcium	0.3 mg
Dietary Fiber	0.0 g

Percent of calories from:

Carbohydrate:	94%
Protein:	6%
Fat:	0%

Pumpkin Pie

Rolling out pastry is often the dreaded task of even the best bakers. Try this fool-proof method to simplify pastry making. With rolling pin, roll pastry out between 2 sheets of waxed paper, rolling away from body and holding waxed paper firmly between counter and stomach. Turn paper as you want to form pastry into circle.

Gently remove top layer of waxed paper; replace. Flip over and remove other piece of paper. Invert 9-inch (23 cm) pie plate onto pastry and flip. Gently remove remaining waxed paper. Ease pastry into pie plate, letting it relax against sides. Crimp edges. Set aside.

Serve this with Yogurt Sauce (page 167) or Vanilla Ice Cream (page 186) for a traditional harvest dessert.

1 cup	all-purpose flour	250 mL
¼ tsp	salt	1 mL
⅓ cup	shortening (at room temperature)	75 mL
3 tbsp	cold water	50 mL

Filling

1	can (14 oz/398 mL) pumpkin purée	1
1 cup	soy milk or lactose-reduced milk	250 mL
2	eggs	2
¾ cup	loosely packed brown sugar	175 mL
2 tbsp	each dark rum and liquid honey	25 mL
1 tsp	each cinnamon and ground ginger	5 mL
½ tsp	ground cloves	2 mL
¼ tsp	each grated nutmeg and salt	1 mL

1. Preheat oven to 425°F (220°C).

2. In mixing bowl, stir together flour and salt. Using pastry blender or 2 knives, cut in shortening until in coarse crumbs. Using fork, stir in water just until pastry sticks together. Form into ball.

3. Roll out pastry. See tip.

4. Filling: In mixing bowl, whisk together pumpkin purée, milk, eggs, brown sugar, rum, honey, cinnamon, ginger, cloves, nutmeg and salt. Pour into pie shell.

5. Bake 20 to 25 minutes or until golden brown. Reduce heat to 350°F (180°C) and continue to bake 25 to 30 minutes or until firm. Cool.

Per serving

Calories	260.7
Protein	4.3 g
Carbohydrate	37.4 g
Fat	9.9 g
Calcium	43.9 mg
Dietary Fiber	1.9 g

Percent of calories from:

Carbohydrate:	56%
Protein:	6%
Fat:	34%

Frozen Delectables

A LIFE without ice cream is unimaginable! A luscious ending to a rich meal or a cooling slurp on a hot day, ice cream is one of life's simple pleasures. With that in mind, it was essential to develop lactose-free ice cream for people with lactose intolerance.

The recipes in this section are not true ice cream, which is normally made by stirring cream into a cooled custard, then freezing it. Instead, these are more like a frozen soufflé. Beaten egg white, instead of cream, is folded into the custard. This method makes a beautifully smooth frozen dessert. It does not require a special ice cream machine but freezes in a shallow pan. It is quick and simple to make with less fat than traditional ice cream made with cream.

The other type of frozen dessert included is sorbet. Although not ice creams but water ices, these particular sorbets have a creamy texture like ice cream due to the smooth texture of the fruit purée used. Enjoy!

Vanilla Ice Cream

The vanilla bean gives the ice cream an intense flavor and a distinctive speckled appearance. Vanilla beans are available in gourmet shops, delicatessens and some bulk food stores.

6	egg yolks	6
⅔ cup	granulated sugar	150 mL
1	vanilla bean	1
½ cup	soy milk or lactose-reduced milk	125 mL
4	egg whites	4
½ tsp	cream of tartar	2 mL

1. In mixing bowl and using electric mixer, beat egg yolks and 1/3 cup (75 mL) of the sugar until thickened and lemony in color, about 2 minutes.

2. With sharp knife, cut vanilla bean in half lengthwise; add to egg yolks along with milk.

3. In heavy stainless steel saucepan, cook yolk mixture, whisking, over medium-low heat until thick enough to coat back of spoon, 5 to 8 minutes. Do not boil. Immediately remove from heat; strain through sieve into bowl. Cover and let cool to room temperature.

4. In clean mixing bowl and using clean beaters on high speed, beat egg whites with cream of tartar until soft peaks form. Gradually beat in spoonfuls of remaining sugar until stiff peaks form.

5. Fold about one-third egg white mixture into cooled custard. Fold in remaining egg whites.

6. Spoon mixture into shallow pan; cover with plastic wrap and freeze 4 hours or overnight. Ice cream can be frozen for up to 2 days.

Makes about 4 cups (1 L), 8 servings

You strain egg mixture through sieve, using the back of a spoon to push through sieve, to ensure a smooth product, removing any lumps caused from curdling.

If you don't have cream of tartar on hand, simply substitute a pinch of salt. Cream of tartar helps stabilize the egg white into firm peaks.

Per serving (1/2 cup/125 mL)

Calories	115.0
Protein	4.1 g
Carbohydrate	15.6 g
Fat	4.1 g
Calcium	18.7 mg
Dietary Fiber	0.2 g

Percent of calories from:

Carbohydrate:	54%
Protein:	14%
Fat:	32%

A glass baking dish or plastic storage container works well for freezing ice cream quickly. Do not use an aluminum container as it may react with the food.

The easiest way to separate eggs is using three bowls. Separate the egg over one bowl, then put the yolk in second bowl and the white in the third bowl. That way if you break a yolk in with the white, you can discard it rather than contaminate the pure yolks and whites. Why so fussy about a little yolk in with the white? Because the egg white will not beat up into stiff peaks if yolk is present.

Any extra egg whites can be frozen for up to 1 month.

Variations:

Lemon: Substitute 1/2 cup (125 mL) fresh lemon juice for the vanilla bean and milk in Step 2. Add 1 tbsp (15 mL) grated lemon rind after straining in Step 3.

Coffee: Substitute 2 tbsp (25 mL) instant coffee granules dissolved in 2 tbsp (25 mL) water for the vanilla bean and milk in Step 2. Add 1 tsp (5 mL) vanilla in Step 5.

Mocha: Substitute 1 cup (250 mL) soy milk or lactose-reduced milk, 1/2 cup (125 mL) unsweetened cocoa powder and 2 tbsp (25 mL) instant coffee granules for the vanilla bean and milk in Step 2; beat until dissolved. Add 1 tsp (5 mL) vanilla in Step 5.

Strawberry: Purée 2 cups (500 mL) fresh or frozen strawberries and substitute for vanilla bean and milk in Step 2.

Mango Sorbet

Be sure to use fully ripe mangoes. Mangoes are ripe when they have a distinct sweet fragrance, deep orange color and feel tender to the touch.

Makes 2 cups (500 mL),
4 servings

3	large mangoes	3
½ cup	each water and granulated sugar	125 mL
¼ cup	fresh lime juice	50 mL

1. Scrape mango flesh away from pit and skin. Purée flesh in food processor using pulsing motion or mash until smooth to make about 1-1/2 cups (375 mL).

2. In saucepan, bring water and sugar to boil; reduce heat and simmer 2 minutes. Let cool to room temperature.

3. Stir lime juice and cooled syrup into mango purée until well combined.

4. Freeze in ice cream maker according to manufacturer's directions or in shallow pan covered with plastic wrap for 4 hours or for up to 2 days.

Per serving (1/2 cup/125 mL)

Calories	201.0
Protein	0.9 g
Carbohydrate	52.5 g
Fat	0.4 g
Calcium	17.8 mg
Dietary Fiber	3.6 g
	(a source)

Percent of calories from:

Carbohydrate:	97%
Protein:	2%
Fat:	2%

Banana Sorbet

Makes about 4 cups (1 L),
8 servings

For best flavor and sweetness, use overripe bananas. This sorbet is so creamy, it's more like ice cream.

To speed cooling of sugar syrup, pour into shallow container and refrigerate 40 to 45 minutes.

3	large bananas	3
¼ cup	fresh lemon juice	50 mL
1 cup	each granulated sugar and water	250 mL

1. Using fork, mash banana or purée in food processor until smooth to make about 1-1/2 cups (375 mL). Add lemon juice; stir or purée to combine.

If you have ripe bananas and aren't ready to use them, pop them into the freezer with the skins on until ready to transform them into sorbet or some other treat. **Peel** while still frozen and defrost a few minutes before mashing.

2. In saucepan, bring water and sugar to boil; reduce heat and simmer 2 minutes. Let cool to room temperature.

3. Stir cooled syrup into banana purée.

4. Freeze in ice cream maker according to manufacturer's directions or in shallow pan covered with plastic wrap for 4 hours or for up to 2 days.

Per serving (1/2 cup/125 mL)

Calories	138.0
Protein	0.5 g
Carbohydrate	35.7 g
Fat	0.2 g
Calcium	3.8 mg
Dietary Fiber	0.8 g

Percent of calories from:
Carbohydrate:	97%
Protein:	1%
Fat:	1%

Apricot Sorbet

For a sophisticated finale, drizzle a spoonful of apricot brandy or orange liqueur over each serving.

Makes about 2 cups
(500 mL), 4 servings

1 cup	dried apricots	250 mL
2 cups	water	500 mL
1 cup	granulated sugar	250 mL
¼ cup	fresh lemon juice	50 mL

1. In saucepan, cover apricots with 1 cup (250 mL) of the water; bring to boil. Reduce heat to medium; simmer until very tender and water has been absorbed, about 5 minutes.

2. Meanwhile, in saucepan, bring remaining water and sugar to boil; reduce heat and simmer 2 minutes. Let cool to room temperature.

3. Purée apricots in food processor along with lemon juice and sugar syrup until smooth. If little bits of fruit remain, this will add texture to the sorbet.

4. Freeze in ice cream maker according to manufacturer's directions or in shallow pan covered with plastic wrap for 4 hours or for up to 2 days.

Per serving (1/2 cup/125 mL)

Calories	290.3
Protein	1.5 g
Carbohydrate	75.5 g
Fat	0.2 g
Calcium	21.8 mg
Dietary Fiber	0.6 g

Percent of calories from:
Carbohydrate:	98%
Protein:	2%
Fat:	1%

Biscuit Tortoni

Makes 8 servings

These dainty Italian confections are ideal for entertaining because they can be made ahead and kept frozen. Look for amaretti biscuits in Italian grocery stores.

Whenever working with eggs, especially if using raw egg white in a dessert, check expiry date on the carton. Discard any eggs with cracks. Always buy them refrigerated and keep them refrigerated. Wash hands thoroughly after separating eggs.

½ cup	chopped unblanched almonds	125 mL
4	egg whites	4
1/4 cup	granulated sugar	50 mL
2 tbsp	amaretto liqueur	25 mL
1 cup	amaretti biscuits	250 mL
½ cup	coarsely chopped drained maraschino cherries (optional)	125 mL
½ tsp	almond extract	2 mL

1. Preheat oven to 350°F (180°C). Toast almonds on baking sheet about 15 minutes or until golden and fragrant. Let cool.

2. In bowl and using electric mixer, beat egg whites until soft peaks form. Gradually beat in sugar until stiff peaks form. Fold in liqueur.

3. In separate bowl and using hands, crush amaretti biscuits to make 1/2 cup (125 mL) coarse crumbs. Reserve half crumbs.

4. Fold crumbs, cherries (if using), cooled almonds and almond extract into egg white mixture. Spoon into 8 large pretty muffin papers or dainty serving cups. Sprinkle with reserved crumbs.

5. Cover with plastic wrap; freeze for 4 hours or for up to 2 days.

Per serving

Calories	173.0
Protein	5.4 g
Carbohydrate	23.8 g
Fat	5.8 g
Calcium	42.9 mg
Dietary Fiber	1.3 g

Percent of calories from:

Carbohydrate:	54%
Protein:	12%
Fat:	30%

Chocolate Lovers

CHOCOLATE CREATES a problem for lactose-intolerant people if it is not pure chocolate. Pure chocolate is lactose-free and can be tolerated, while milk chocolate or chocolate products containing milk can cause lactose-intolerance symptoms.

Cocoa, like chocolate, is made from the cocoa bean but without the cocoa butter contained in chocolate. It has several advantages in baking: it's easier to use than chocolate because it can be stirred into mixtures without melting; it's fat free; and it has a full flavor. Best of all, cocoa contains no lactose.

Fudge Pudding

Serve this hot and comforting self-saucing pudding with Vanilla Ice Cream (page 186) or Yogurt Sauce (page 167) if yogurt is tolerated.

Makes 6 servings

1 cup	all-purpose flour	250 mL
½ cup	granulated sugar	125 mL
¼ cup	unsweetened cocoa powder	50 mL
1 tsp	each baking soda and baking powder	5 mL
¼ tsp	each cinnamon and salt	1 mL
1½ tsp	instant coffee granules	7 mL
½ cup	hot water	125 mL
2 tbsp	vegetable oil	25 mL

If you prefer, use fresh double-strength perked coffee rather than instant coffee dissolved in hot water.

Sauce

¼ cup	packed brown sugar	50 mL
¼ cup	unsweetened cocoa powder	50 mL
¼ cup	currants, rinsed	50 mL
1 tbsp	dark rum	15 mL
1 tbsp	instant coffee granules	15 mL
1½ cups	boiling water	375 mL

1. Preheat oven to 350°F (180°C). Grease 6-cup (1.5 L) baking dish.

2. In mixing bowl, stir together flour, sugar, cocoa, baking soda, baking powder, cinnamon and salt. Dissolve instant coffee in hot water (or use 1/2 cup/ 125 mL strong fresh-perked coffee); stir into dry mixture along with oil. Spread in prepared dish.

3. Sauce: In mixing bowl, stir together sugar, cocoa, currants and rum. Dissolve instant coffee in boiling water (or use 1-1/2 cups/375 mL strong fresh-perked coffee); gradually whisk into bowl. Pour over batter in dish.

4. Bake for 40 to 45 minutes or until bubbly and cake has risen to top.

Per serving
(with sauce)

Calories	249.7
Protein	3.9 g
Carbohydrate	49.0 g
Fat	5.5 g
Calcium	37.0 mg
Dietary Fiber	1.2 g

Percent of calories from:

Carbohydrate:	73%
Protein:	6%
Fat:	18%

*C*hocolate Mousse

Rich with cream and eggs, chocolate mousse is a classic finale to a special dinner. This recipe is lactose-free but has all the same rich flavor. Without the cream, it is lower in fat too!

To toast almonds, spread on baking sheet and bake in preheated 350°F (180°C) oven about 15 minutes or until golden brown and fragrant.

¾ cup	granulated sugar	175 mL
½ cup	unsweetened cocoa powder	125 mL
¼ cup	water	50 mL
1 tbsp	instant coffee granules	15 mL
5	eggs, separated	5
¼ tsp	salt	1 mL
2 tbsp	Grand Marnier	25 mL
¼ cup	sliced toasted almonds	50 mL

1. In saucepan, stir together sugar, cocoa, water and coffee granules; cook over medium heat, stirring frequently, until smooth and thickened, 3 to 4 minutes.

2. Beat egg yolks; whisk into cocoa mixture and cook about 1 minute. Let cool.

3. Meanwhile, in separate mixing bowl, beat egg whites with salt until stiff peaks form. Stir Grand Marnier into cooled cocoa mixture. Fold in egg whites.

4. Spoon into glass dishes, demitasse cups or wine glasses. Sprinkle with toasted almonds. Refrigerate until serving time or for up to 1 day.

Per serving

Calories	225.0
Protein	7.3 g
Carbohydrate	33.3 g
Fat	8.3 g
Calcium	62.5 mg
	(a source)
Dietary Fiber	1.0 g

Percent of calories from:

Carbohydrate:	54%
Protein:	12%
Fat:	30%

Cappuccino Cookies

Originally, these were a buttery shortbread-like cookie but shortening with added flavoring makes a good substitute for butter to produce a melt-in-your-mouth cookie that's rich in flavor.

Makes 4 dozen cookies

The baked cookies freeze well in freezer containers, or the raw dough may be frozen ready to bake into cookies.

2½ cups	cake-and-pastry flour	625 mL
½ cup	unsweetened cocoa powder	125 mL
1 tsp	cinnamon	5 mL
½ tsp	salt	2 mL
1 tbsp	each instant coffee granules and vanilla	15 mL
1 cup	each granulated sugar and packed brown sugar	250 mL
1 cup	shortening	250 mL
1	egg	1

1. Preheat oven to 350°F (180°C). Line baking sheet with parchment paper.

2. In mixing bowl, stir together flour, cocoa, cinnamon and salt; set aside. In separate bowl, dissolve coffee in vanilla; set aside.

3. In another bowl and using electric mixer, beat together 3/4 cup (175 mL) of the granulated sugar, all the brown sugar, shortening and egg until fluffy. Gradually beat in flour mixture and coffee mixture until it starts to hold together.

4. Divide mixture into 48 equal portions. Place remaining granulated sugar in small bowl; roll each portion in sugar to coat, making 1-inch (2.5 cm) balls.

5. Arrange cookies on prepared baking sheet, leaving 1-inch (2.5 cm) space between each. Bake about 20 minutes or until firm to touch.

Fudge Cake

Makes 12 servings

Birthdays in our house would not be complete without this cake. Spread with Cappuccino Sauce (page 209) and serve with an accompanying bowl of sauce for both the cake and one of the ice creams (pages 186-87). It's a winning combination.

This cake freezes well for six months, although you will have to wrap it well so that no one knows what is inside!

2 cups	all-purpose flour	500 mL
¾ cup	unsweetened cocoa powder	175 mL
2 tsp	baking powder	10 mL
1 tsp	baking soda	5 mL
1 tsp	cinnamon	5 mL
½ tsp	salt	2 mL
1½ cups	granulated sugar	375 mL
¾ cup	shortening	175 mL
3	eggs	3
1 tbsp	instant coffee granules	15 mL
1¼ cups	warm water	300 mL
1 tsp	vanilla	5 mL

1. Preheat oven to 350°F (180°C). Line 9-inch (2.5 L) springform pan with parchment paper.

2. In large bowl, sift together flour, cocoa, baking powder, baking soda, cinnamon and salt.

3. In separate bowl with electric mixer, beat sugar and shortening until fluffy. Beat in eggs one at a time, until well combined. Dissolve coffee in warm water.

4. Beat flour mixture and coffee alternately into shortening mixture. Stir in vanilla. Spoon evenly into prepared pan.

5. Bake for 55 to 65 minutes or until toothpick inserted in centre comes out clean. Let cool in pan 10 minutes. Run knife around edge of pan; remove cake and discard paper. Let cool on racks.

Per serving (1/12th)
(without sauce)

Calories	378.9
Protein	5.6 g
Carbohydrate	60.4 g
Fat	15.3 g
Calcium	41.0 mg
	(a source)
Dietary Fiber	0.8 g

Percent of calories from:

Carbohydrate:	60%
Protein:	6%
Fat:	34%

Cheesecake

OBVIOUSLY A traditional cheesecake requires cream cheese and often sour cream—both definite noes for lactose-intolerant people. However, silken soft or firm tofu provides calcium and makes a low-fat, lactose-free substitute for creaminess and texture. If you don't believe me, try these recipes and taste for yourself! You won't be disappointed.

Lemon Cheesecake

Makes 8 servings

One of my favorite desserts, this New York-style cheesecake uses tofu to replace the usual cream. Try it with a spoonful of Quick Strawberry or Blueberry Sauce (page 208).

1½ cups	graham wafer crumbs	375 mL
¼ cup	granulated sugar	50 mL
3 tbsp	vegetable oil	50 mL
1 tsp	cinnamon	5 mL

To prevent a metallic taste, line pan with parchment paper. This way, the acid from the filling cannot react with the metal pan.

Filling

2	pkg (each 10.5 oz/297 g) silken firm tofu	2
4	eggs, separated	4
1 cup	granulated sugar	250 mL
¼ cup	fresh lemon juice	50 mL
2 tbsp	all-purpose flour	25 mL
1 tbsp	grated lemon rind	15 mL
1 tsp	vanilla	5 mL
½ tsp	salt	2 mL

1. Preheat oven to 350°F (180°C).

2. Using sieve, drain tofu.

3. In mixing bowl, stir together graham wafer crumbs, sugar, oil and cinnamon. Press onto bottom and 1 inch (2.5 cm) up sides of 9-inch (2.5 L) springform pan. Bake for 10 minutes. Let cool.

4. In food processor, beat together drained tofu, egg yolks, sugar, lemon juice, flour, lemon rind, vanilla and salt until smooth.

5. In separate bowl and using electric beaters, beat egg whites until stiff. Fold into lemon mixture. Turn into prepared shell.

6. Bake for 60 to 65 minutes or until almost firm in center. Cool before cutting into wedges to serve.

Per serving

Calories	357.2
Protein	9.3 g
Carbohydrate	53.0 g
Fat	12.6 g
Calcium	47.2 mg
Dietary Fiber	0.1 g

Percent of calories from:

Carbohydrate:	59%
Protein:	10%
Fat:	31%

Amaretto Cheesecake

Silken firm tofu makes a good substitute for cream cheese in this delicate almond cheesecake. It may be made up to one day ahead.

Makes 8 servings

1 cup	vanilla wafer crumbs	250 mL
¼ cup	granulated sugar	50 mL
¼ cup	sliced toasted almonds	50 mL
2 tbsp	vegetable oil	25 mL
¼ tsp	almond extract	1 mL

Filling

2	pkg (each 10.25 oz/297 g) silken firm tofu	2
½ cup	granulated sugar	125 mL
⅓ cup	amaretto liqueur	75 mL
1 tsp	grated lemon rind	5 mL
2	eggs	2
¼ cup	sliced almonds	50 mL

1. Preheat oven to 350°F (180°C). Spray 10-inch (25 cm) pie plate with nonstick baking spray.

2. Using sieve, drain tofu.

3. In mixing bowl, stir together vanilla wafer crumbs, sugar, almonds, oil and almond extract. Press onto bottom and up side of pie plate.

4. In food processor, purée together drained tofu, sugar, amaretto, lemon rind and eggs until smooth. Pour into prepared pie plate. Sprinkle almonds on surface around edge. Bake for 50 to 55 minutes or until firm.

Per serving	(1/8th)
Calories	308.1
Protein	9.3 g
Carbohydrate	36.5 g
Fat	13.2 g
Calcium	68.3 mg
	(a source)
Dietary Fiber	1.4 g

Percent of calories from:

Carbohydrate:	46%
Protein:	12%
Fat:	37%

Raspberry Cheesecake in a Glass

Makes 10 servings

Similar to a Bavarian cream but lower in fat than the traditional one made with whipping cream, this tofu version has a full, rich fruit flavor once it is well chilled and set.

3	pkg (each 10.25 oz/290 g) silken soft tofu	3
1	pkg (1 tbsp/15 mL) unflavored gelatin	1
1	can (300 mL) undiluted raspberry juice concentrate	1
⅓ cup	granulated sugar	75 mL
2 tsp	vanilla	10 mL
	Fresh raspberries	

1. Using sieve, drain tofu.

2. In small saucepan, sprinkle gelatin over 1/2 cup (125 mL) of the raspberry concentrate. Let stand 10 minutes. Heat over low heat, stirring, until gelatin dissolves, 2 to 3 minutes.

3. In food processor, purée together drained tofu, remaining raspberry concentrate, sugar and vanilla until smooth. With motor running, pour in dissolved gelatin through feed tube. Purée until well combined.

4. Pour about 1/2-cup (125 mL) servings into dainty serving bowls. Refrigerate at least 4 hours or for up to 2 days. Serve with a sprinkling of fresh raspberries.

Per serving

Calories	98.4
Protein	4.9 g
Carbohydrate	14.1 g
Fat	2.6 g
Calcium	27.5 mg
Dietary Fiber	0.0 g

Percent of calories from:

Carbohydrate:	57%
Protein:	20%
Fat:	24%

Tiramisu

The Italian version of trifle, tiramisu is typically made with a high-fat soft cheese called mascarpone—definitely not on the food list for lactose-intolerant people! Once again, silken soft tofu comes to the rescue as a substitute in this creamy confection.

Serves 8

2	pkg (each 10.25 oz/290 g) silken soft tofu	2
5	egg yolks	5
½ cup	granulated sugar	125 mL
½ cup	dark rum	125 mL
3	egg whites	3
Pinch	salt	Pinch
½ cup	hot water	125 mL
1 tbsp	instant coffee granules	15 mL
1	pkg (7 oz/200 g) ladyfingers	1
¼ cup	unsweetened cocoa powder	50 mL

1. Using sieve, drain tofu.

2. In deep mixing bowl with electric mixer, beat egg yolks, sugar and 1/4 cup (50 mL) of the rum until thickened, 3 to 4 minutes.

3. In heavy saucepan over medium heat, cook egg yolk mixture, whisking to prevent curdling, until thick enough to coat back of spoon, about 5 minutes. Do not boil. Cool. Strain through sieve.

4. Meanwhile, in clean bowl and using clean beaters, beat egg whites with salt until stiff peaks form. Set aside.

5. In food processor or blender, purée drained tofu. Add rum custard and combine. Remove to clean bowl; fold in beaten egg white.

6. In small bowl, mix hot water with instant coffee to dissolve; stir in remaining rum. Dip ladyfingers into coffee mixture; arrange some in bottom of glass bowl. Spread with about one-third rum custard; arrange some ladyfingers in single layer on top. Spread another third of custard on top of ladyfingers; top with remaining ladyfingers. Spread with remaining rum custard. Sift cocoa over entire dessert.

7. Cover and refrigerate up to 1 day in advance.

Per serving

Calories	266.9
Protein	8.6 g
Carbohydrate	32.3 g
Fat	7.2 g
Calcium	51.4 mg
Dietary Fiber	0.0 g

Percent of calories from:

Carbohydrate:	48%
Protein:	13%
Fat:	24%

*C*hocolate Cheesecake Squares

Individual pieces can be picked up and enjoyed with a good cup of coffee.

Makes 16 squares

1 cup	graham wafer crumbs	250 mL
2 tbsp	granulated sugar	25 mL
2 tbsp	vegetable oil	25 mL
½ tsp	cinnamon	2 mL

Chocolate Filling

1	pkg (10.25 oz/290 g) silken soft tofu	1
⅔ cup	granulated sugar	175 mL
⅓ cup	unsweetened cocoa powder	75 mL
2 tsp	vanilla	10 mL
½ tsp	salt	2 mL
2	eggs	2
	Sliced strawberries (optional)	

1. Preheat oven to 350°F (180°C). Line 8-inch (2 L) square cake pan with parchment paper.

2. Using sieve, drain tofu.

3. In mixing bowl, stir together graham wafer crumbs, sugar, oil and cinnamon. Press onto bottom of pan.

4. In mixing bowl using electric mixer, beat together drained tofu, sugar, cocoa, vanilla, salt and eggs until smooth. Pour into prepared pan.

5. Bake for 35 to 40 minutes or until firm. Cool on rack. Cut into 16 equal squares. Garnish each piece with strawberry slice (if using).

Per serving	(1/16th)
Calories	106.6
Protein	2.3 g
Carbohydrate	16.4 g
Fat	3.9 g
Calcium	14.2 mg
Dietary Fiber	0.0 g

Percent of calories from:

Carbohydrate:	59%
Protein:	8%
Fat:	32%

Sauces, Fillings and Toppings

Amaretto Cream

Use this cream as a dip for fruit or as a sauce for desserts to replace whipping cream.

1	pkg (10.25 oz/290 g) silken soft tofu	1
¼ cup	granulated sugar	50 mL
3 tbsp	amaretto liqueur	45 mL
½ tsp	grated lemon rind	2 mL

1. Using sieve, drain tofu.

2. In food processor, purée drained tofu, sugar, amaretto and lemon rind until smooth. Pour into serving bowl. Cover and refrigerate for up to 4 hours.

Per serving (2 tbsp/25 mL)

Calories	49.3
Protein	1.4 g
Carbohydrate	7.5 g
Fat	0.8 g
Calcium	8.3 mg
Dietary Fiber	0.0 g

Percent of calories from:

Carbohydrate:	59%
Protein:	11%
Fat:	15%

Vanilla Cream Filling

Makes about 1 cup
(250 mL)

This cream and its flavorful variations can be used for dessert toppings, cake toppings or tart fillings. Try them with pancakes or crêpes.

⅓ cup	granulated sugar	75 mL
2 tbsp	cornstarch	25 mL
¼ tsp	salt	1 mL
1 cup	lactose-reduced milk	250 mL
1	egg	1
1 tsp	vanilla	5 mL

1. In saucepan, whisk together sugar, cornstarch and salt.

2. Gradually whisk in lactose-reduced milk, egg and vanilla. Cook over medium heat, whisking frequently, until smooth and thickened, about 5 minutes.

3. Remove from heat; cover surface directly with plastic wrap. Let cool. Cream can be refrigerated for up to 2 days or frozen up to 1 month. Stir before using.

Variations:

Coffee Cream Filling: Stir 2 tsp (10 mL) instant coffee granules into 1 cup (250 mL) hot water; use instead of lactose-reduced milk.

Chocolate Cream Filling: Add 3 tbsp (50 mL) unsweetened cocoa powder to dry ingredients. Substitute soy milk for lactose-reduced milk if desired.

Mocha Cream Filling: Add 1 tbsp (15 mL) unsweetened cocoa powder to dry ingredients. Dissolve 1 tbsp (15 mL) instant coffee granules in 1 cup (250 mL) water or lactose-reduced milk; use instead of lactose-reduced milk.

Per serving (2 tbsp/25 mL)

Calories	62.8
Protein	1.7 g
Carbohydrate	11.0 g
Fat	1.3 g
Calcium	41.7 mg
Dietary Fiber	0.0 g

Percent of calories from:

Carbohydrate:	71%
Protein:	11%
Fat:	19%

Quick Strawberry Sauce

This instant sauce always brings back happy memories of picking berries under a sunny sky—one of my favorite pastimes! It is perfect as a topping for ice creams, Orange Pancakes (page 76), Yeast Blini (page 78) or Currant Scones (page 145).

Makes about 2 cups
(500 mL)

4 cups	whole strawberries	1 L
1 cup	granulated sugar	250 mL
2 tbsp	cornstarch	25 mL
1 tsp	grated orange rind (optional)	5 mL

Frozen berries work equally well in this recipe.

1. In saucepan, stir together strawberries, sugar, cornstarch and orange rind (if using).

2. Bring to boil over high heat; reduce heat to medium-low and simmer, stirring until thickened, about 5 minutes. (Mixture will thicken more after cooling.)

3. Spoon into jar; cover and refrigerate up to 2 weeks.

Variation:
Quick Blueberry Sauce: Substitute blueberries for strawberries. Substitute lemon rind for orange rind.

Per serving   (2 tbsp/25 mL)

Calories	62.8
Protein	0.2 g
Carbohydrate	15.9 g
Fat	0.1 g
Calcium	5.2 mg
Dietary Fiber	0.8 g

Percent of calories from:

Carbohydrate:	97%
Protein:	1%
Fat:	2%

*C*appuccino Sauce

Makes about 1⅓ cups
(325 mL)

Keep a jar of this versatile sauce in your refrigerator to serve over ices, drizzle over cake, use as a dip for fresh fruit or to stir into soy milk or lactose-reduced milk for hot cocoa.

¾ cup	unsweetened cocoa powder	175 mL
¾ cup	granulated sugar	175 mL
1 tbsp	instant coffee granules	15 mL
1 tsp	vanilla	5 mL
1	cinnamon stick	1
Pinch	salt	Pinch
1 cup	hot water	250 mL

1. In saucepan, stir together cocoa, sugar, coffee granules, vanilla, cinnamon stick and salt.

2. Place over medium heat, gradually whisk in hot water until smooth. Cook, stirring, until thickened, about 5 minutes. Discard cinnamon stick. Cool.

3. Pour into jar; cover and refrigerate up to 2 weeks.

Per serving (2 tbsp/25 mL)

Calories	72.9
Protein	1.3 g
Carbohydrate	18.9 g
Fat	0.6 g
Calcium	11.5 mg
Dietary Fiber	0.1 g

Percent of calories from:

Carbohydrate:	87%
Protein:	6%
Fat:	6%

Old-Fashioned Chocolate Sauce

For those with lactose intolerance, combining chocolate sauce with hot lactose-reduced milk makes a delicious calcium-rich drink. If you are just getting used to the taste of soy milk, try mixing it with this chocolate sauce. Remember that although soy milk is nutritious, it is not a calcium source like cow's milk.

Makes about ⅔ cup
(150 mL)

To make hot cocoa, stir 2 tsp (10 mL) chocolate sauce into 1 cup (250 mL) milk. Cook in saucepan, frequently stirring, over medium heat about 4 minutes or just until it starts to bubble. Pour into mug and serve.

½ cup	unsweetened cocoa powder	125 mL
½ cup	granulated sugar	125 mL
½ cup	hot water	125 mL
2 tsp	instant coffee granules	10 mL
1 tsp	vanilla	5 mL

1. In saucepan, whisk together cocoa and sugar. Gradually whisk in water, coffee and vanilla until smooth. Cook, stirring often, over medium heat about 5 minutes or until glossy and thickened.

2. Pour into jar; cover and refrigerate for up to 2 weeks.

Per serving (2 tbsp/25 mL)

Calories	40.8
Protein	0.7 g
Carbohydrate	10.5 g
Fat	0.3 g
Calcium	6.1 mg
Dietary Fiber	0.0 g

Percent of calories from:

Carbohydrate:	88%
Protein:	6%
Fat:	6%

Appendix I

Celebration Menus

Typically, North American celebrations are full of rich food dressed in buttery sauces with a creamy dessert to finish. I hope these menu ideas will help those planning a lactose-free event to make it as much a celebration for lactose-intolerant people as it is for everyone else.

Adult Birthday Dinner

This menu is ideal for a simple yet tasty summer birthday barbecue. It is particularly appealing to men and teens who enjoy these robust tastes.

FILET MIGNON: Instead of usual garlic butter, rub the steak with a clove of garlic, grind fresh pepper over and brush with extra virgin olive oil before grilling. Serve with a horseradish sauce.

> Caesar Salad with Creamy Garlic Dressing (page 51)
>
> Baked Potatoes with Tofu Sour Cream (page 127)
>
> Tomato Basil Salad (page 63, margin)
>
> Fudge Cake with Ice Cream (page 197, 186)

A Child's Birthday Party

Preparing a children's party can be an intimidating experience. Children let you know if they like something or not. Over the years, I have found that putting out a selection of foods for them to make their own works well. You control what is put out on trays, and they control what they eat. The only item that is fully prepared is the fruit punch, which always seems to be a hit.

VEGGIES AND DIP: Put out a selection of crudités. Make sure you include carrots, because they are usually the most popular. My choice for dip would be something relatively plain. Most kids love garlic: use the Creamy Garlic Caesar Salad Dressing (page 51) or the basic Tofu Cream (page 50).

MAKE-YOUR-OWN PITAS: Put out a basket of pitas, cut in half for easy stuffing, along with bowls of shredded lettuce, grated carrot, sliced cucumber, pickles, sunflower sprouts, chopped egg, tuna salad and shredded smoked chicken.

DECORATED CUPCAKES: Using the Basic Sponge (page 180) or Fudge Cake (page 197) recipe, pour batter into colorful paper liners. Preheat oven to 350°F

(180°C); bake for 20 to 25 minutes or until firm to touch and toothpick inserted in center comes out clean. Put out trays of cupcakes with bowls of Chocolate Sauce (page 210) or Lemon Butter (page 166) to dip cupcakes into. Set out bowls with sugar-based candies like jubejubes or sprinkles for the kids to decorate their cakes. Do not include chocolate candies like Smarties® because they contain lactose.

FRUIT PUNCH: Somehow a fruit punch is always special. Cranberry-raspberry mixed with ginger ale, or peach cocktail with ginger ale, are two popular combinations although lemonade always seems to work well too. Float some strawberries, sliced oranges, lemon or limes on top to make it look festive.

Thanksgiving

Herb Roasted Turkey (page 106)
Loaf Pan Carrot Stuffing (page 107)

CREAMY SWEET POTATOES: Cook the potatoes in water until tender and mash with a little orange juice and brown sugar. An electric mixer works well to make them smooth and creamy. Season to taste with salt and pepper.

GREEN BEANS WITH ALMONDS: Cook the beans in boiling salted water. Drain. Toss with about 1 tbsp (15 mL) extra virgin olive oil and a squeeze of lemon. Give this vegetable dish a calcium boost with a sprinkling of toasted almonds. Toast unblanched almonds in a preheated 350°F (180°C) oven about 15 minutes; chop coarsely. Just before serving sprinkle over beans.

Pumpkin Pie with Vanilla Ice Cream (page 186)

Christmas

The Christmas season is always a hectic time of year, but this streamlined menu allows the chief cook time off to enjoy the day, since everything except for turkey can be done in advance. Even the turkey is a lazy cook's dream.

Salted Almonds (page 28)
Herb Roasted Turkey (page 106)
Loaf Pan Stuffing (page 107)
Carrot Squash Crumble (page 118)
Mashed Potato Casserole (page 117)
Lactose-free Shortbread (page 179)
Chocolate Yule Log (page 181)

Easter

BAKED HAM: Ham is lactose-free providing the glaze chosen contains no milk products. A simple glaze of honey mustard is delicious. Bake according to directions on the label.

Scalloped Potatoes (page 119)

Carrots with Maple Syrup (page 120)

Spring Salad with Oriental Flavors (page 65)

Lemon Torte made from Basic Meringue (page 182) spread with Lemon Butter (page 166)

Putting on the Ritz

Artichokes with Spicy Lemon Sauce (page 121)

Grilled Salmon (page 112)

Salad of Spring Greens, New Potatoes and Asparagus (page 64)

Jelly Roll made from Basic Sponge (page 181) and spread with Lime Butter (page 166, variation)

Appendix II

NUTRIENT ANALYSIS

The nutrient analysis done on the recipes in this book is derived from the following databases:

Canadian Nutrient File 1991, USDA Handbook #8, and finally, when those two sources are not suitable, manufacturer's information.

Recipes are evaluated as follows:

When there is a range of servings, the smaller of the two numbers and therefore the larger portion is selected.

When optional ingredients are listed, they are not evaluated.

When salt, pepper or icing sugar is not quantified, it is not calculated in the recipe.

When a choice is given for ingredients, for example, honey or corn syrup, only the first is used in the calculation.

Recipes listing variations are evaluated only for the basic or initial recipe.

Terminology:

CALCIUM CLAIMS: "a source" = 55 mg to 164 mg
"a high source" = 165 mg to 274 mg
"a very high source" = 275 mg and higher

DIETARY FIBRE CLAIMS: "a source" = at least 2 g per serving
"a high source" = at least 4 g per serving
"a very high source" = at least 6 g per serving

NOTE: Numbers for "percentage of calories from" may not always total 100 due to rounding or because elements in addition to carbohydrate, protein and fat make up the total.

Index